POINT-OF-CARE
GLUCOSE DETECTION FOR
DIABETIC MONITORING
AND MANAGEMENT

POINT-OF-CARE GLUCOSE DETECTION FOR DIABETIC MONITORING AND MANAGEMENT

Sandeep Kumar Vashist

Chief Scientific Officer, Vallo Med Health Care, Germany

John H.T. Luong

Walton fellow (Science Foundation of Ireland) and Professor,
Department of Chemistry at University College Cork, Ireland

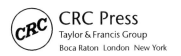

CRC Press
Taylor & Francis Group
Boca Raton London New York

CRC Press is an imprint of the
Taylor & Francis Group, an **informa** business

CRC Press
Taylor & Francis Group
6000 Broken Sound Parkway NW, Suite 300
Boca Raton, FL 33487-2742

First issued in paperback 2020

© 2017 by Taylor & Francis Group, LLC
CRC Press is an imprint of Taylor & Francis Group, an Informa business

No claim to original U.S. Government works

ISBN 13: 978-0-367-57405-5 (pbk)
ISBN 13: 978-1-4987-8875-5 (hbk)

Visit the Taylor & Francis Web site at
http://www.taylorandfrancis.com

and the CRC Press Web site at
http://www.crcpress.com

Contents

Preface

The word diabetes is from Latin, meaning 'siphon', itself derived from the Greek for 'pass through', as the patient passes too much water (polyuria). This term originates from Aretus the Cappadocian, a Greek physician practising in the second century AD. English doctor Thomas Willis added 'mellitus' to the term in 1675 to indicate excess glucose in urine. Mel is 'honey' in Latin, and so diabetes mellitus is defined as 'siphoning off sweet water'. As also reported in ancient China, ants were attracted to diabetic patients' urine since it was sweet. Glucose is a principal source of energy for the human body, but it needs to be regulated to avoid hyperglycaemia or hypoglycaemia. In the past, diabetes was a feared disease and eventually led to death with multi-organ damage and painful complications. The journey of insulin discovery, a silver bullet for diabetic management and control, began with two brilliant Canadian scientists who later shared a Nobel Prize in medicine. Unfortunately, diabetes has become an unsustainable economic burden as this global epidemic has increased at an unprecedented pace; in 2015 it affected some 415 million people worldwide. Although there is no cure for diabetes, those living with the disease can still enjoy a full and satisfying life provided they know how to manage their glucose levels by balancing diet with exercise and medicine, if necessary. Insulin and over 40 drugs are available for the treatment of both type 1 and type 2 diabetes.

This book describes the role of point-of-care (POC) glucose monitoring as an essential part of diabetes management to regulate blood glucose levels within their normal physiological range.

Thanks to advanced medicine, clinical chemistry, modern biology, powerful electronics and miniaturisation technology, compact medical devices for monitoring glucose with high precision, excellent sensitivity and reliability are commercially available. The current generation of blood glucose monitoring devices (BGMD) in the form of glucose meters are truly advanced devices with the desired attributes of precision, accuracy, robustness, connectivity, simplicity and cost-effectiveness. Some of the systems, including the FreeStyle Libre of Abbott, are remarkable as they have obviated the use of lancets and test strips and enable continuous glucose monitoring for two weeks. Also of note is the advent of iHealth Align, the world's smallest smartphone-based blood glucose meter that has ushered in a revolutionary era of personalised mobile healthcare. Similarly, considerable advances have been made in continuous and non-invasive glucose monitoring (NGM) systems. The monitoring of glycated haemoglobin (HbA1c) has also become an underlying trend in diabetic healthcare.

OBJECTIVES OF THE BOOK

This book aims to present the field of POC glucose monitoring, which is a critical requirement for diabetic healthcare monitoring and management. The various POC glucose monitoring technologies and devices are described in comprehensive detail together with their characteristics, pros and cons, and potential roles in diabetic management.

SCOPE

We describe POC glucose monitoring based on BGMD, continuous glucose monitoring systems (CGMS), NGM devices, and HbA1c monitoring devices. There is an in-depth description of various glucose monitoring technologies and methods together with the principle of detection, advantages, limitations/pitfalls, device characteristics and diagnostic performance.

TARGET AUDIENCE

We aim to provide a thorough understanding and comprehensive view of the field of POC glucose monitoring to healthcare professionals, biomedical engineers/scientists, researchers, healthcare economists, policy makers, investors, professionals in preventive healthcare, and persons interested in personalised healthcare. It also serves as a very useful resource and teaching aid for professionals and researchers in diabetic monitoring and management, preventive healthcare, medicine, bioengineering, mobile healthcare, science, and research.

ORGANISATION

The text encompasses the key themes of POC glucose monitoring for diabetic management. The first chapter provides an overview of the diabetes epidemic and the need for POC glucose measurement. Chapter 2 focuses on BGMD with recent developments and advances in the field of blood glucose meters together with challenges and future trends. Subsequently, the NGM technologies and devices are discussed in the third chapter, providing details of various NGM principles along with their limitations and prospects. The fourth chapter covers the bioanalytical performance, principles of operation, advantages, potentials, limitations and future trends of continuous glucose monitoring systems. Chapter 5 discusses the critical need for analysis of HbA1c as a biomarker for the long-term average of blood glucose level in a diabetic. Different analytical methods are described together with commercial devices and POC assays for the quantitative determination of HbA1c. Chapter 6 looks at the continuous improvement in diabetes management software that enables easy analysis, trend prediction, better data visualisation, and safe and secure data storage. Also discussed are smart applications that are providing an efficient universal platform for diabetic management with improved mobile health and telemedicine tools. Chapter 7 addresses the issue of analytical and clinical accuracy of SMBG and whether improvement in analytical accuracy would lead to improved clinical outcomes for patients. The final chapter draws the threads of the book together, with concluding remarks.

Apart from its critical importance in diabetic healthcare monitoring and management, glucose is an important indicator in persons with impaired glucose tolerance (IGT), who are at a high risk of developing diabetes in the near future. Moreover, it is a useful metabolite in the general population, which will be helpful for personalised preventive healthcare. The monitoring of glucose will enable the screening and identification of persons affected by IGT and diabetes, which is one of the primary goals in tackling diabetes, considering the 48% rate of undiagnosed diabetic cases worldwide.

The knowledge and insight provided in this book for POC glucose monitoring will enable more effective diabetic management and the development of critically improved devices equipped with personalised mobile healthcare for next-generation diabetes care.

POC testing plays an instrumental role in improving access to medical procedures for early detection, diagnosis, and treatment. The implementation of new portable and accessible devices will lead to improved health technologies.

Sandeep Kumar Vashist
Melbourne, Australia
John HT Luong
Cork, Ireland

Contributors

Sandeep Kumar Vashist, Micro/Nanophysics Research Laboratory, Royal Melbourne Institute of Technology, 124 La Trobe Street, Melbourne, VIC 3124, Australia and Vallo Med Health Care GmbH, Castrop-Rauxel, Germany

John HT Luong, Innovative Chromatography Group, Irish Separation Science Cluster (ISSC), Department of Chemistry and Analytical, Biological Chemistry Research Facility (ABCRF), University College Cork, Cork, Ireland

Peter B Luppa, Institute of Clinical Chemistry and Pathobiochemistry, Klinikum rechts der Isar der Technische Universität München, Ismaninger Str. 22, D-81675 Munich, Germany

Erwin Schleicher, Department of Internal Medicine, Division of Clinical Chemistry/Central Laboratory, University of Tübingen, Hoppe-Seylerstr. 3, D-72076, Tübingen, Germany

Albert Donald Luong, Cleveland Clinic, 2950 Cleveland Clinic Blvd, Weston, FL 33331, United States

CHAPTER 1

Diabetes: a growing epidemic and the need for point-of-care testing

Sandeep Kumar Vashist and John HT Luong

CHAPTER SUMMARY

Diabetes has been declared as a global epidemic and emergency by the International Diabetes Federation (IDF), as the current incidence level has surpassed all previously projected numbers. Indeed, it has reached a catastrophic level, which substantiates the need for all essential steps for more effective diagnosis, monitoring, and management. The diabetic patient needs to perform continual monitoring of blood glucose, followed by intervention and management to cope with this disease. Ideally, the current high cost of consumables and miniaturised blood glucose meters (BGMs) must be reduced significantly, particularly for patients in developing nations. Continuous glucose monitoring systems offer the potential for real-time monitoring of glucose levels. However, current non-invasive glucose monitoring (NGM) technologies have not matched the desired clinical accuracy to replace the BGM. Together with advanced optical methods, the ongoing trend towards smartphone-based mobile healthcare is further facilitating the monitoring of physical activity and basic healthcare parameters, which contributes to the prevention, or delays the onset, of this debilitating disease.

Keywords: diabetes; glucose; point-of-care testing; blood glucose meters; non-invasive glucose monitoring devices; continuous glucose monitoring systems.

CONTENTS

INTRODUCTION

Diabetes is a global emergency and the topmost concern for governments and public health authorities worldwide.[1] The unprecedented increasing incidence during the last decade together with the unsustainable economic burden substantiates the need for taking all essential measures to suppress its further growth. In general, insulin deficiency and its associated glucose disorder can be attributed to diabetic consequences. A total lack of insulin is referred to as type 1 diabetes, which was formerly called juvenile onset or insulin-dependent diabetes. Endocrine pancreas cells, spreading over the pancreas surface like small islands, produce insulin, glucagon, and other hormones. They are known as islets of Langerhans, after the pathologist who discovered these islet cells. In type 1, the body's immune system destroys the islet, which eventually eliminates the synthesis of insulin. Thus, cells cannot absorb sugar (glucose), which they need to produce energy. Type 1 might account for 5 to 10 out of 100 diabetic patients. In type 2 diabetes, the level of insulin is low or the patients cannot use insulin effectively, and this accounts for the vast majority of people who have diabetes, 90–95%. As type 2 diabetes progresses, the pancreas may make less and less insulin; that is, insulin deficiency, whereas insulin resistance is referred to as the state where the body is unable to use insulin. Type 2 diabetes (adult onset or non-insulin-dependent diabetes) can develop at any age but becomes more apparent during adulthood. However, an increasing number of children are being diagnosed with the disease. Type 1 cannot be prevented, while type 2 can be prevented or delayed with a healthy diet and physical activity. Even with proper treatment, diabetes remains the leading cause of blindness and kidney failure, a critical risk factor for heart disease, stroke, and foot or leg amputations. There is a severe form of diabetes, known as brittle diabetes, which is characterised by increasing and decreasing blood sugar levels at rapid rates. Brittle diabetes is almost exclusive to type 1 diabetes (also called a subtype of type 1 or diabetes complication); however, people with type 2 diabetes are not immune to this glucose fluctuation.

Point-of-care testing (POCT) is the only option for diabetics to check their blood glucose levels and fluctuation. Patients can then keep their blood glucose levels within the desired physiological range by dietary and healthcare interventions. Otherwise, subsequent life-threating diabetic complications are unavoidable, which account for significant healthcare costs. A wide range of POC glucose monitoring devices has been developed such as BGMs, NGM devices and CGMS. The most widely used devices are the BGMs, while CGMS are more appropriate for those who require continuous glucose monitoring (CGM). Although various NGM devices and concepts have been developed, a clinically precise and robust NGM device has not been achieved so far. This chapter provides an overview of diabetes and the POCT of glucose.

GLUCOSE AND INSULIN RELATIONSHIP

Human beings require about 160–200 g of glucose per day as an energy source for cellular metabolism and brain functions. Indeed, two-thirds of glucose (about 100–130 g) is specifically needed by the brain to cover its high energy requirements. As a dense network of neurons, or nerve cells, which are constantly active, the brain depends on a continuous supply of glucose from the bloodstream. After food ingestion, glucose is absorbed and released into the bloodstream by the small intestine and the stomach. Glucose per se cannot penetrate into the cells directly and thus circulates in the bloodstream. Beta cells, the predominant type of cells in the islets of Langerhans, are sensitive to glucose levels and regulate the pancreas to release insulin, corresponding to the blood glucose level. Insulin is then secreted into the blood where it travels throughout the body and helps regulate blood sugar. Beta cells also secrete amylin and C-peptide together with insulin. Thus, beta cells in the pancreas play three important tasks: producing, storing and releasing the hormone insulin. Insulin attaches itself to the insulin receptor (IR), a transmembrane receptor, resulting in an 'open' channel that allows the passage of glucose. The IR belongs to the large class of tyrosine kinase receptors and is activated by insulin and free insulin-like growth factors (IGF-I and IGF-II). A 'substrate' protein that is phosphorylated by the insulin receptor is known as IRS-1 (insulin receptor substrate 1). IRS-1 binding and phosphorylation lead to an increase in the high-affinity glucose transporter (Glut4) molecules on the outer membrane of insulin-responsive tissues, including muscle cells and adipose tissue. Glut4 is transported from cellular vesicles to the cell surface, where it then can mediate the transport of glucose into the cell. Indeed, insulin plays three important roles: (i) it helps muscle, fat, and liver cells absorb glucose from the bloodstream, lowering blood glucose levels, (ii) it stimulates the liver and muscle tissue to store excess glucose as glycogen, and (iii) it lowers blood glucose levels by reducing glucose production in the liver.

Insulin is a peptide, consisting of 51 amino acids in two peptide chains. Preproinsulin is the primary translational product of the insulin gene, a biologically inactive precursor of insulin. This 110 amino acid peptide is converted into proinsulin by signal peptidases, which remove its signal peptide from its N-terminus. Proinsulin is then converted into the bioactive hormone insulin by removal of the C-peptide. In addition, amylin, a 37 residue peptide hormone, is co-secreted with insulin (1:100 ratio) from the pancreatic beta cells, which are also deficient in diabetic people. Amylin inhibits glucagon secretion, delays gastric emptying and acts as a satiety agent. It acts as a short-term regulator of blood glucose level by diminishing the rate of glucose entering the bloodstream. The C-peptide helps to prevent neuropathy and other vascular complications by assisting in the repair of the arterial muscular layers. Insulin stimulates glycogen synthesis and inhibits glycogen breakdown.

In contrast, glucagon, a peptide hormone produced by alpha cells of the pancreas, raises the concentration of glucose in the bloodstream. Its effect is opposite to that of insulin, which lowers the glucose. The pancreas A cells release glucagon when the concentration of glucose in the bloodstream falls too low. Glucagon binds to the glucagon receptors of the liver and causes it to convert stored glycogen, which is released into the bloodstream. Thus, glucagon and insulin are part of a feedback system that keeps blood glucose levels at a stable level (Fig. 1.1).

About 5% of people, particularly children and young adults, have type 1 diabetes as their bodies cannot produce insulin because their body's immune system (i.e. white blood cells called T cells) attacks and destroys the beta cells. Unfortunately, type 1 diabetes is not diagnosed until all beta cells have already been destroyed. Consequently, a person with type 1 depends on insulin to survive. Insulin itself may be a key trigger of the immune attack on beta cells because antibodies to insulin and other proteins produced by beta cells are found in people with type 1 diabetes. Researchers test for these antibodies to help identify people at increased risk of developing the disease.

Testing the types and levels of antibodies in the blood can help determine whether a person has type 1 diabetes or latent autoimmune diabetes of adults (LADA), a slow onset type 1 diabetes, or another type of diabetes.

In type 2 diabetes, the body does not use insulin properly; that is, there is insulin resistance. For a short term, the insulin resistance can be overcome as the pancreas will make extra insulin for glucose regulation. However, in the long term, the pancreas cannot make enough insulin, and elevated glucose level begins its detrimental effects on the body if not regulated by drug intervention or insulin injection. Both type 1 and type 2 diabetes result from a complete or partial loss of beta cell number and function. Based on the role of insulin and glucagon in glucose regulation, the drugs designed for diabetes target the secretion of insulin or depression of glucagon to maintain the glucose level within the acceptable range (Table 1.1)

After subcutaneous insulin injection, the period it takes for the insulin to be absorbed and start lowering the blood glucose is the *onset* time. For some time, the total insulin activity will increase and cause blood glucose to decrease. As more of the insulin is absorbed and starts to be effective, the total insulin activity gets higher and reaches its maximum (the *peak* activity time), corresponding to the minimal blood sugar level. As the insulin is metabolised by the body, the total insulin activity decreases and the blood glucose starts to increase

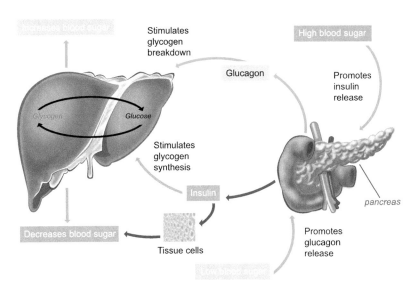

FIGURE 1.1 Relationship of blood glucose, insulin, and glucagon. (The illustrations of the liver and pancreas are from Google Images.)

TABLE 1.1 Some drugs for the treatment of diabetes and their mechanisms

Type 2 DM-drugs	Side effects	General description
Metformin (Glucophage)	Diarrhoea, nausea, and abdominal pain. Low risk of developing low blood sugar.	The first-line oral medication for the treatment of type 2 diabetes, particularly for gestational diabetes. It is generally well tolerated. However, it is not for patients with liver disease or kidney problems. Metformin decreases glucose production by the liver and increases glucose use by body tissues.
Second-generation sulfonylureas (SUs). • First-generation SUs include long-acting chlorpropamide, tolbutamide, tolazamide, and acetohexamide. • Second-generation SUs include glyburide (glibenclamide), glipizide, gliquidone, and glimepiride, which vary the duration of action. • Glimepiride and glyburide are longer acting agents than glipizide. • Glimepiride (pictured, right) is the newest second-generation SU or a third-generation SU. It has larger substitutions than other second-generation SUs.	It should be used with caution with the elderly and in patients with renal or hepatic disease.	Only the second generation of SUs is allowed. All first-generation drugs were discontinued. The drug promotes the release of insulin from pancreas beta cells. It reduces fasting plasma glucose, postprandial glucose, and glycosylated haemoglobin levels. It is a useful and cost-effective drug.

Type 2 DM-drugs	Side effects	General description
Thiazolidinediones (TZD) or Glitazones • Troglitazone (Rezulin, Resulin, Romozin, Noscal). 	TZD is associated with increased risks of cardiac failure, cardiovascular events, and hip fractures (USFDA warning). Pioglitazone (Actos) is suspended in France and Germany due to the risk of bladder cancer. Rezulin was withdrawn due to an increased incidence of drug-induced hepatitis.	TZDs stabilise the beta cells in the pancreas in the production of insulin to stop the development of DM. It has been suggested that TZDs activate a receptor common in fat cells, nuclear peroxisomal proliferator-activated receptors gamma (PPAR-gamma). Thus, the uptake or absorption of fat cells is increased, the metabolism of glucose is increased, and the liver's production of new glucose is reduced. Pioglitazone is used alone or in combination with metformin or a sulfonylurea such as glyburide.
DPP-4 (gliptins) • Inhibitors of dipeptidyl peptidase 4) • Sitagliptin (Januvia). • Janumet (combined sitagliptin and metformin). • Juvisync (combined sitagliptin and simvastatin – a lipid-lowering medication)	No harmful effect of DPP-4 inhibitors on all-cause mortality, cardiovascular mortality, or stroke. It might cause an increase in heart failure, but the statistics are only marginally significant. Fewer side effects, less hypoglycaemia and less weight gain. It is often combined with other drugs. Its efficacy is challenged.	DPP-4 inhibitors reduce glucagon and blood glucose levels. The mechanism of DPP-4 inhibitors is to increase incretin levels (glucagon-like peptide-1 and gastric inhibitory polypeptide), which inhibit glucagon release, which in turn increases insulin secretion.

again. The total amount of time that the insulin is active is called the *duration*. The pattern of onset, peak, and duration is sometimes called the activity profile.

DIABETES: FACTS AND FIGURES

As the commonest non-communicable disease, diabetes has been declared a global epidemic by IDF[1] and World Health Organization (WHO). The last two decades have witnessed an unprecedented increase in diabetic cases. The number of diabetics, as estimated by WHO in 2004,[2] was expected to rise from 171 million in 2000 to 366 million by 2030 (Table 1.2). However, there were already 382 million diabetics in 2013,[3] reflecting its unprecedented growth. The current estimate of 415 million diabetes by IDF (Fig. 1.2) might rise to 642 million by 2040[1] (Fig. 1.3A). This clear trend, adding over 8 million new diabetics every year, demands immediate counteractive measures, which is the paramount healthcare concern globally for effective diabetic management. There are also an estimated 192.8 million undiagnosed diabetic cases that account for a large number of diabetics progressing towards lethal diabetic complications entirely unnoticed.[1] Additionally, about 318 million people with impaired glucose tolerance (IGT) (Fig. 1.3B), characterised by high blood glucose, have a high risk of developing type 2 diabetes mellitus during their life[1] due to the underutilisation of insulin, whereas type 1 is the underproduction of insulin by insulin-producing beta cells in the pancreas.

Population-based studies have consistently shown that most of the persons with diabetes had never been diagnosed with the disease in their early years. The *IDF Diabetes Atlas* (2015)[1] conveys a strong message about a worrying indication of the future impact of diabetes as a major threat to global development. This is a wake-up call for all nations to take strong initiatives and actions to tackle this most challenging health problem of the 21st century. In brief, diabetes

TABLE 1.2 Continuously increasing the incidence of diabetes

	2004 by WHO[2]	2013 by IDF[3]	2015 by IDF[1]
Number of diabetics	2000 – 171 M	2013 – 382 M	2015 – 415 M
Predicted number of diabetics	2030 – 366 M	2035 – 592 M	2040 – 642 M

M = million

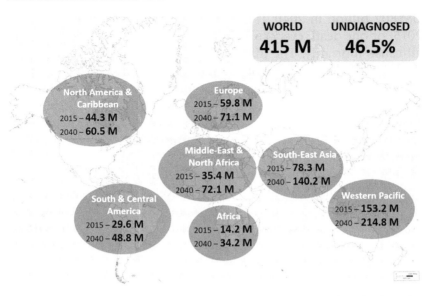

FIGURE 1.2 Prevalence of diabetes worldwide at present and projections for 2040. (Statistics from *IDF Diabetes Atlas*, 7th ed., 2015 by IDF.[1])

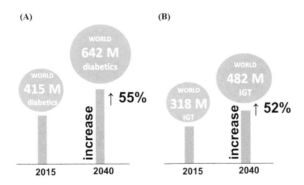

FIGURE 1.3 Prevalence of (A) diabetes and (B) IGT at present and projections for 2040. (Statistics from *IDF Diabetes Atlas*, 7th ed., 2015 by IDF.[1])

carries an unsustainable economic burden regarding persistently high healthcare costs; greater care and financial support desired from family members/carers; loss of workplace productivity; and disability. Both acute and long-term complications result from diabetes such as hypoglycaemia, ketoacidosis, amputations, coma, neuropathy, and retinal damage.

The health spending on diabetes accounted for 11.2% of global health expenditure in 2015, or US$673 billion, and might reach

US$802 billion in 2040[1] (Fig. 1.4A). It caused 5 million deaths in 2015, or one death every six seconds, accounting for 8.4% of global all-cause mortality. The diabetes mortality is, in fact, more than the combined mortalities of several infectious diseases: HIV/AIDS (1.5 million), malaria (0.6 million), and tuberculosis (1.5 million)[1] (Fig. 1.4B). However, the actual mortality rate, which is hard to evaluate due to diabetic complications, is very high. It can account for 50% or more of deaths due to cardiovascular disease, a major diabetic complication. Another most worrying factor is the approximately 46.5% of cases of undiagnosed diabetics worldwide, which has quite a similar level of incidence in developed as well as developing nations (Fig. 1.5). This demands communal screening strategies based on POCT that can provide adequate diagnosis of such undiagnosed diabetic cases.

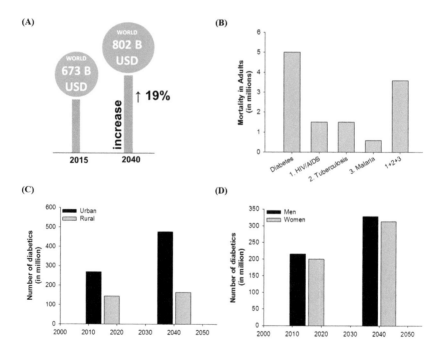

FIGURE 1.4 (A) Healthcare spending on diabetes at present and projections for 2040. (B) Mortality due to diabetes in comparison to that of HIV/AIDS, tuberculosis, and malaria (individual and combined). (C) Prevalence of diabetes in urban and rural settings at present and projections for 2040. (D) Prevalence of diabetes in men and women today and projections for 2040. (Statistics from *IDF Diabetes Atlas*, 7th ed., 2015 by IDF.[1])

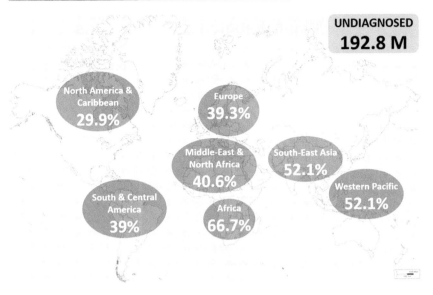

FIGURE 1.5 Prevalence of undiagnosed diabetics worldwide at present. (Statistics from *IDF Diabetes Atlas*, 7th ed., 2015 by IDF.[1])

Type 2 diabetes accounts for 85–95% of all diabetes in high-income countries and even higher in low- and middle-income countries. Rapid cultural and social changes, increasing urbanisation, change in diet, ageing populations, unhealthy behaviour and reduced physical activities are collectively attributed to this substantial increase. These factors contribute to the increased prevalence of diabetes in urban settings compared to rural settings (Fig. 1.4C). Similarly, it is slightly more prevalent in men than women (Fig. 1.4D). About 80% of diabetics live in low- and middle-income countries, where healthcare spending on diabetes is the least. A person with type 2 diabetes can live for several years without any symptoms, which results in a silent body damage and associated diabetic complications such as retinopathy, nephropathy, chronic kidney disease, and heart failure (Fig. 1.6). Other medical problems associated with diabetes mellitus include anxiety disorders, celiac disease (digestive disorder), depression, and mood and eating disorders. Therefore, the earlier a person is diagnosed with diabetes and monitoring and management begins, the better are the chances of preventing late-stage diabetes with harmful and costly diabetic complications. This substantiates the need for robust and reliable POCT devices for the efficient management of diabetes and for timely intervention. The existing diabetic BGM market is US$13 billion, almost double from $US8.8 billion in 2008.[4] However,

Major diabetes complications

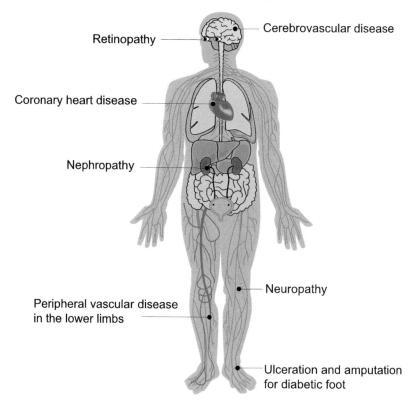

FIGURE 1.6 Major complications associated with diabetes mellitus. (Illustration from www.imhealth.com/diabetes-complications/. Reproduced with permission from IMHealth.com.)

as the number of IGT individuals is quite close to the number of diabetics, the POCT can cater to a substantially higher market size.

POC glucose monitoring is a critical requirement for diabetics, which enables them to live a healthy lifestyle, obviating the costly late-stage diabetic complications that account for 73% of diabetic healthcare management costs. The early-stage diagnosis of diabetes will significantly add to life expectancy and improve the quality of life. Patients can prevent or delay the onset of diabetes by making a simple and low-cost lifestyle change or nutritional/healthcare intervention. The steadily increasing diabetic population in each nation poses a big threat to society as it is an unbearable economic burden draining most of the healthcare resources for the continuous monitoring and management of diabetics. The early disability from diabetes further places a heavy and debilitating burden not only on the affected persons and their families but also eventually on the society and the nation. The diabetics, particularly at an advanced stage, require constant healthcare monitoring and management, including dieting and physical activities, which significantly affect their work performance, thereby resulting in a decrease in productivity. Moreover, patients have a direct impact on their family members and relatives, whose lives are adversely affected due to associated healthcare costs, and the care and attention that they need to provide to the diabetic(s). The continuous exposure of family members to increased psychological stress might also lead to depression or anxiety.

POINT-OF-CARE GLUCOSE MONITORING

BGMs are the most widely used and accepted POCT devices for monitoring glucose levels, using a low-cost test strip and a simple electrochemical reaction.[5] There are considerable advances in such electrochemical biosensors, categorised as the first, second and third generations, with glucose oxidase (GOx) as the biorecognition element (Table 1.3). However, they require finger pricking using the standard lancing device to withdraw a blood sample of a few microlitres. In addition, electrochemical biosensing is still subject to significant interference caused by the following United States Food and Drug Administration (FDA) listed chemicals[6]: acetaminophen, salicylic acid, tetracycline, dopamine, ephedrine, ibuprofen, L-DOPA, methyl-DOPA, tolazamide, ascorbic acid, bilirubin, cholesterol, creatinine, triglycerides, and uric acid.

During the last two decades, there have been significant improvements in the blood glucose sensing chemistries, calibration, miniaturisation, mediators, response time, sample volume, robustness, and precision. The current generation of BGMs is further equipped with advanced device features such as internal memory, multi-user functionality, wireless transmission, diabetic management software, integral storage of various test strips, prediction of trends and alarm alerts. The commercialisation of iHealth Align, the smallest FDA-approved smartphone-based BGM by iHealth (USA), is the next-generation POCT device, which employs a miniaturised blood glucose sensing dongle that plugs directly into the 3.5 mm audio jack of a smartphone.

Although the BGMs have high precision, they still require finger pricking, which is problematical for long-term monitoring of this disease, particularly with infants. There have been continual efforts by several companies and researchers to arrive at a prospective NGM device[6] that alleviates the pain and suffering of diabetics, thereby enabling more frequent monitoring. However, none of the NGM devices has shown the same high analytical precision as BGMs, which is the main reason these devices have not become commercially viable. Nevertheless, a wide range of potential NGM technologies has been demonstrated in recent years with some innovative devices including MediWise (UK) that are currently under evaluation.

The need for CGMS has been widely supported by numerous clinical findings.[7] A wide range of such commercial POCT devices has already been launched successfully. However, they are only being used by a limited number of diabetics. Doubtlessly, NGM-based CGMS would be an ideal POCT device for diabetics, which would motivate the users to monitor frequently their glucose levels and keep them within the acceptable physiological range.

The current advances in cellphone (CP) based technologies[8-10] and the upcoming smart watches, equipped with personalised healthcare monitoring of basic physiological health parameters, will be a definite asset to diabetics if they can also perform the NGM. This trend is one of the main objectives for ongoing developments in smart and wearable technologies for personalised mobile healthcare (mH).

OTHER SHORT-TERM GLYCAEMIC INDICATORS

Besides the measurement of blood glucose, serum 1, 5-anhydroglucitol (1, 5-AG) has been used for monitoring short-term glycaemic control in Japan under the name GlycoMark™ for almost two decades. This indicator represents diabetic status over a 24-hour period to reflect glucose's competitive inhibition of 1,5-AG reabsorption in the kidney tubule.[11] In brief, AG is a naturally occurring monosaccharide found in most foodstuffs. Blood AG decreases during times of hyperglycaemia and returns to normal levels after approximately two weeks in the absence of hyperglycaemia. Thus, it can be used for people with type 1 or type 2 diabetes to trace a history of high blood glucose where current glycaemic measurements of HbA1c and blood glucose monitoring show normal values.

The enzymatic colorimetric assays can be implemented with materials from GlycoMark Inc. (Winston-Salem NC) and Kyowa Medex (Tokyo, Japan). The GlycoMark assay is based on a reagent mixture, consisting of glucokinase, pyruvate kinase, and phosphoenol pyruvate, which converts endogenous glucose to glucose-6-phosphate. Pyranose oxidase is added to oxidise AG to produce hydrogen peroxide, which can be determined by different procedures. In the Kyowa Medex assay, AG is converted to 1, 5-anhydro-glucitol-6-phosphate (AG-6-P) by adenosine-5'-diphosphate (ADP)-dependent hexokinase and ADP. AG-6-phosphate dehydrogenase reacts with AG-6-P and β-NADP$^+$, producing β-NADPH. Diaphorase (DIP) promotes the reaction of NADPH and 2-(4-iodophenyl)-3-(4-nitrophenyl)-5-(2, 4-disulfo-phenyl)-2H-tetrazolium sodium to produce a water-soluble formazan pigment with an absorbance at 450 nm. Despite this possible use and the approval of the GlycoMark assay by the FDA, the AG test is not common. It is not suitable for monitoring gestational diabetes as renal haemodynamics is not stable during pregnancy.

Apolipoprotein B is another short-term marker, a component of glycated low-density lipoproteins (LDLs), which might be involved in atherogenesis. Considering the 3–5-day circulating half-life of LDLs, the glycated LDL level indicates mean glycaemia of the previous week.[12] The average concentration of glycated LDL from non-diabetic subjects is 21.8 ± 0.9 mg/L (3.35% of total apolipoprotein B), compared to 40.8 ± 2.6 mg/L (9% of total apolipoprotein B) of patients with type 2 diabetes.[13] Despite the potential importance of glycated LDL in atherosclerosis associated with diabetes, there is no suitable method for its determination in the clinical setting. Nevertheless, monoclonal antibodies, designated ES12, can recognise glycated apolipoprotein B epitopes in the LDL complex in human plasma

TABLE 1.3 Advances in the development of electrochemical biosensors for glucose measurement

Generation	Principles and features
First generation	The reduced GOx (FADH$_2$) is converted back to the oxidised form by the sample dissolved oxygen. The by-product of this enzymatic reaction, H$_2$O$_2$ can be determined by electrochemical oxidation or reduction.
Second generation	The oxidation of the reduced GOx is achieved by a small mediator with ferrocene or its derivatives. The redox property of such mediators can be followed and related to the glucose level.
Third generation	The FAD redox cofactor of GOx is covalently or electrochemically anchored on the working electrode to facilitate the rapid oxidation and reduction of the enzyme in the presence of oxygen.
Fourth generation	Direct electron transfer (DET), i.e. the reduced GOx (FADH$_2$) is re-oxidised to GOx (FAD). Both nanowiring and nanomaterials play an important role in DET.

and such antibodies have been used in a competitive enzyme-linked immunosorbent assay (ELISA) to measure glycated LDL concentrations in plasma.[13] Note also that glycated LDL is more prone to *in vitro* oxidation and has a different electrophoretic mobility, compared to native LDL.[14] This feature can be exploited in capillary electrophoresis to discriminate glycated LDL from its native counterpart.

CONCLUSIONS

The uncontrolled increase in the number of diabetics worldwide and the growing healthcare spending on diabetes cannot be sustained for long. Therefore, effective strategies are required to combat the further increase in diabetes. The constant improvements in BGMs and the evolving CGMS have led to considerable improvements in diabetic monitoring and management. The new developments and ongoing efforts in NGM devices are further providing the hope of painless glucose monitoring devices, which will lead to critically improved diabetic healthcare. The upcoming trend in personalised mobile healthcare using smartphones and smart watches are further providing the impetus for the development of wearable smart NGM devices for POC glucose monitoring.

Nanomaterials such as graphene, carbon nanotubes, nanocomposites and the like could improve sensor performance, biocompatibility in the case of implanted sensors, and stimulation of blood flow with biocoating materials to shorten the lag time between interstitial fluid (IF) glucose concentrations and blood glucose.

REFERENCES

1. International Diabetes Federation. *IDF Diabetes Atlas*, 7th ed. www.diabetes atlasorg/resources/2015-atlashtml#. 2015.
2. Wild S, Roglic G, Green A, Sicree R, King H. Global prevalence of diabetes: estimates for the year 2000 and projections for 2030. *Diabetes Care*. 2004; 27(5): 1047–53.
3. *IDF Diabetes Atlas*, 6th ed. www.idforg/sites/default/files/EN_6E_Atlas_ Full_0pdf. 2013.
4. Hughes MD. The business of self-monitoring of blood glucose: a market profile. *J Diabetes Sci Technol*. 2009; 3(5): 1219–23.
5. Vashist SK, Zheng D, Al-Rubeaan K, Luong JHT, Sheu FS. Technology behind commercial devices for blood glucose monitoring in diabetes management: a review. *Anal Chim Acta*. 2011; 703(2): 124–36.
6. Vashist SK. Non-invasive glucose monitoring technology in diabetes management: a review. *Anal Chim Acta*. 2012; 750: 16–27.

7. Vashist SK. Continuous glucose monitoring systems: a review. *Diagnostics.* 2013; 3(4): 385–412.

8. Vashist SK, Luppa PB, Yeo LY, Ozcan A, Luong JHT. Emerging technologies for next-generation point-of-care testing. *Trends Biotechnol.* 2015; 33(11): 692–705.

9. Vashist SK, Mudanyali O, Schneider EM, Zengerle R, Ozcan A. Cellphone-based devices for bioanalytical sciences. *Anal Bioanal Chem.* 2014; 406(14): 3263–77.

10. Vashist SK, Schneider EM, Luong JHT. Commercial smartphone-based devices and smart applications for personalized healthcare monitoring and management. *Diagnostics.* 2014; 4(3): 104–28.

11. Buse JB, Freeman JL, Edelman SV, Jovanovic L, McGill JB. Serum 1, 5-anhydroglucitol (GlycoMark™): a short-term glycemic marker. *Diabetes Technol Ther.* 2003; 5(3): 355–63.

12. Lyons TJ, Baynes JW, Patrick JS, Colwell JA, Lopes-Virella MF. Glycosylation of low density lipoprotein in patients with type 1 (insulin-dependent) diabetes: correlations with other parameters of glycaemic control. *Diabetologia.* 1986; 29(10): 685–9.

13. Cohen MP, Lautenslager G, Shea E. Glycated LDL concentrations in non-diabetic and diabetic subjects measured with monoclonal antibodies reactive with glycated apolipoprotein B epitopes. *Eur J Clin Chem Clin Biochem.* 1993; 31(11): 707–13.

14. Sobal G, Menzel J, Sinzinger H. Why is glycated LDL more sensitive to oxidation than native LDL? A comparative study. *Prostaglandins Leukot Essent Fatty Acids.* 2000; 63(4): 177–86.

CHAPTER 2

Blood glucose monitoring devices

Sandeep Kumar Vashist and John HT Luong

CHAPTER SUMMARY

Blood glucose monitoring devices (BGMD) have been significantly improved during the last few decades, enabling more efficient diabetic monitoring and management. The current generation of BGMD equipped with miniaturised test strips and advanced features provides rapid response, high specificity and improved calibration using a simplified measurement procedure. Both analytically superior chemistries and better test strip design enable the processing of a minimal sample, which results in a painless sample uptake. The devices have powerful internal memory, wireless and Cloud connectivity, multiuser support, and integrated diabetic software management. This chapter provides an overview of the developments in BGMD along with the prospects and the growing trend towards wearable BGMD and mobile healthcare.

Keywords: blood glucose monitoring devices; diabetes management; electron mediators; glucose-limiting membranes; interferences; glucose strips.

CONTENTS

INTRODUCTION

Glucose is a primary source of cellular energy, which needs to be tightly regulated by the human body via metabolic homeostasis. The failure to control blood glucose levels leads to *diabetes mellitus*, which is characterised by persistently high levels of blood glucose above the normal physiological range of 4–8 mM (i.e. 72–144 mg dL^{-1}). Type 1 diabetes mellitus occurs when the pancreas does not produce sufficient insulin to regulate the high blood glucose level, whereas type 2 diabetes mellitus manifests when the body is unable to use the secreted insulin. Diabetes damages the blood vessels and nerves and increases the risk for depression, metabolic disorders, and cardiovascular diseases. Diabetes also increases the risk for low testosterone and depression, both of which can contribute to suppressing sexual activities. Despite significant advances in the field and extensive research efforts, a cure for diabetes has not yet been discovered. Therefore, diabetes can only be managed by more frequent blood glucose monitoring (BGM)[1-6] using a commercially available BGMD and keeping the blood glucose level within the normal physiological range. Accordingly, diabetics can sustain a healthy lifestyle and prevent or delay the onset of costly and lethal diabetic complications such as kidney damage, retinopathy, cardiovascular disorders, etc.

BGMD comprises a test strip, which is inserted into a miniaturised handheld glucose meter to effect a rapid electrochemical reaction of glucose with the enzyme coated on the test strip. It requires only minimal whole blood sample (microlitres), which is taken by piercing the fingertip with a painless minimally invasive lancing device.

BGM has been the most extensively studied and investigated field of point-of-care testing (POCT) in diabetic monitoring and management, as evident from the numerous peer-reviewed articles published on this theme during the last two decades (Fig. 2.1). The BGMD, accounts for 85% of the total biosensors market with a present value of US$13 billion. This number reflects an exponential increase from the BGMD market of US$5 billion in 2004.[7] This substantial increase can be attributed to the unprecedented rise in the number of diabetics, improved healthcare facilities, growing awareness and continuously decreasing costs of BGMDs. The need for continuous innovation and support is enormous. Therefore, the commercially viable BGMD are mainly developed and marketed by selected industrial giants such as Roche Diagnostics, Abbott, Bayer, Minimed, Dexcom, and LifeScan. The performance of BGMD has been critically investigated and frequently reviewed.[8–14] The BGMD technologies have been steadily improved in terms of precision, accuracy, cost-effectiveness, miniaturisation, connectivity, readout and other features. This chapter highlights the significant advances in BGMD along with the trend

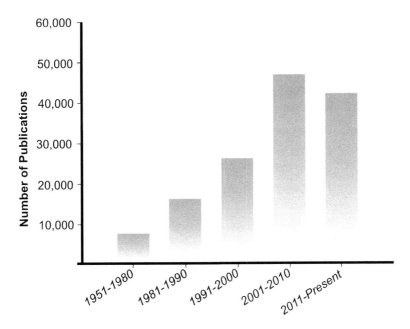

FIGURE 2.1 Total peer-reviewed papers published in the field of blood glucose monitoring during the stated period. (Data from www.sciencedirect.com using 'blood glucose monitoring' in the advanced search option, retrieved 16 March 2016.)

TABLE 2.1 Main events in the history of BGM

Timeline	Main event
1920s	Canadian Frederick Banting and Charles Best determined glucose in blood and urine by analytical methods.
1962	Clark and Lyons developed first glucose biosensor.[15]
1967	Updike and Hicks determined glucose in various biological fluids using an oxygen electrode onto which glucose oxidase (GOx) was immobilised in a gel.[16]
1971	A.H. Clemens from Miles Laboratories, USA (presently part of Bayer) developed the first BGMD, the Ames Reflectance meter, a costly and bulky device.[17]
1975	The YSI glucose analyser was developed by Yellow Springs Instrument Company, USA. It detects glucose based on the amperometric detection of hydrogen peroxide using a platinum electrode and GOx contained within an outer polycarbonate membrane and an inner cellulose acetate membrane. The various models developed to date by the company are being used as standards in clinical analysis.
1987	MediSense (previously Genetics International) introduced an amperometric blood glucose sensor in collaboration with Cranfield and Oxford universities.
1987	Abbott introduced ExacTech, a pen and a strip-based glucose meter (GM). The strip consisted of GOx and a ferrocene-mediated mediator.[18]
1987	LifeScan introduced a test strip design in a One Touch® GM. The strip was made up of a flat piece of plastic, having a hole that was covered by a membrane.
1987 onwards	GM was developed by several companies.
1996	The MediSense blood glucose sensor was acquired by Abbott for US$867 million.
1996	TheraSense Inc. was cofounded by Adam Heller and his son Ephraim Heller.
1998	Roche Diagnostics was formed when Roche merged with Boehringer Mannheim.
1999	TheraSense introduced a thin-layer microcoulometer, which critically reduced the sample required for a blood glucose test to just 300 nL, which led to its use in Abbott's FreeStyle™ BGM.
2001	LifeScan took the BGM technology from Inverness Medical Technology for US$1.3 billion stock-for-stock transactions.
2004	Abbott acquired TheraSense Inc. for US$1.26 billion, which became a part of Abbott Diabetes Care.

Timeline	Main event
2004	The screen-printing based method was developed and used for the mass production of glucose sensing strips.[19] Various inks based on carbon, nanomaterials and nanocomposites have also been developed for use in screen-printing.[20]
2007	The FreeStyle Navigator CGMS was introduced by Abbott Diabetes Care, based on the concept of wired-enzyme.
2014	Abbott introduced the FreeStyle Libre® flash glucose monitoring system,[21,22] which enabled continuous glucose monitoring without any need for test strips, lancets or calibration.
2014	iHealth Labs, Inc. introduced a smartphone-interfaced iHealth glucose monitoring system.
2015	iHealth Labs, Inc. launched the world's smallest US Food and Drug Administration (FDA)-approved smartphone-based GM, iHealth Align.

towards next-generation wearable BGMD equipped with personalised mobile healthcare (mH) tools.

The most important events in the history of BGM are summarised in Table 2.1. BGM started in the 1920s with the development of the analytical methods for BGM, followed by the development of a prospective electrochemical glucose analyser in 1975. Subsequently, the blood glucose meter (GM) was developed along with the test strip design in 1987. The pen-shaped GM was launched in 1990, which resulted in the development and commercialisation of many critically improved mobile-shaped GMs by numerous companies. In the early 21st century, the screen-printing method enabled mass production of test strips. The initiation of continuous glucose monitoring systems (CGMS) was followed by closed-loop systems. The most recent development is the smartphone-based BGMS while the future trend is inclined strongly towards wearable technologies-based non-invasive continuous monitoring systems. A summary of the characteristics of commercial BGMS is given in Table 2.2.

COMPONENTS OF BLOOD GLUCOSE MONITORING DEVICES
Enzymes

GOx and glucose dehydrogenase (GDH), belonging to the family of oxidoreductases, are the two most widely used enzymes in the test strips that enable highly specific detection of glucose. GOx is highly stable and can withstand the harsh ambient conditions prevalent during manufacture and operation. It is isolated from *Aspergillus niger* as a 160 kDa dimeric protein with each monomer having an identical polypeptide chain. The reactive site of each subunit contains flavin adenine dinucleotide (FAD), which is a redox cofactor that gets oxidised by the oxidizing substances such as dioxygen (O_2) by accepting electrons from glucose. The reaction involves sequentially the reaction of FAD-GOx with glucose (equation 1), the oxidation of $FADH_2$-GOx, and the production of H_2O_2 (equation 2). The oxidation of H_2O_2 is directly proportional to the number of blood glucose molecules, thereby enabling its quantification. As a thick protein layer surrounding the FAD at the reactive site limits the direct electron transfer between the GOx reactive site and the electrode, there is a need for the mediator to re-oxidise the GOx-$FADH_2$. Different attempts with considerable success have been reported to overcome the long distance between the redox-active cofactor and the electrode surface, including the use of carbon nanotubes and graphene.[23] Again, dissolved oxygen in the whole blood competes with the electrode for the GOx ($FADH_2$), resulting in an underestimated glucose concentration.

GDH, belonging to the class of quinoproteins, is a homodimeric enzyme, where each monomer binds to a pyrroloquinoline quinone (PQQ) molecule and three calcium ions.[20] It acts as a cofactor to convert glucose to gluconolactone,[24,25] but the oxidation of glucose by GDH is similar to that of FAD-GOx[26] except that the reduced form ($PQQH_2$-GDH) is not oxidised by O_2[26,27] (equations 1–4). The amino acid sequence of GDH from *Bacillus megaterium* has been deciphered, consisting of 4 identical subunits, each containing 262 amino acid residue.[24] A calcium ion activates the PQQ cofactor while the others are needed for the functional dimerisation of GDH.

$$\text{Glucose} + \text{FAD} - \text{GOx} \rightarrow \delta - \text{Gluconolactone} + \text{FADH}_2 - \text{GOx} \qquad (1)$$

$$\text{FADH}_2 - \text{GOx} + \text{O}_2 \rightarrow \text{FAD} - \text{GOx} + \text{H}_2\text{O}_2 \qquad (2)$$

$$\text{FAD} + 2\text{H}^+ + 2\text{e}^- \rightarrow \text{FADH}_2 \qquad (3)$$

$$\text{PQQ} + 2\text{H}^+ + 2\text{e}^- \rightarrow \text{PQQH}_2 \qquad (4)$$

FAD-GOx is highly specific to glucose[28] and is prone to substantial interference by mannose[29] while PQQ-GDH has similar specificity for glucose and maltose.[30] The electron transfer turnover rates of FAD-GOx is $5000\,\text{s}^{-1}$ at 35°C as compared to $11,800\,\text{s}^{-1}$ for PQQ-GDH.[31] Similarly, the apparent reduction potential of FAD-GOx is $-0.048\,\text{V}$ vs standard hydrogen electrode (SHE) at 25°C in the physiological medium at pH 7.2[32] as compared to $10.5 \pm 4\,\text{mV}$ vs SHE for PQQ-GDH at pH 7.0 in the presence of excess Ca^{2+}.[33] Nicotinamide adenine dinucleotide (NAD)- and FAD-dependent GDH enzymes are used in various commercial test strips such as Abbott's Optium™ (NAD-GDH) and Bayer's Contour™ TS (FAD-GDH). They are highly specific for glucose and independent of O_2, but xylose may interfere with the specific glucose detection of NAD-GDH.[34] However, FAD-GDH may react non-specifically with some non-glucose sugars (maltose, mannose, galactose and lactose) that are usually found in persons taking specific medications.[35] Therefore, non-glucose sugars can give falsely elevated glucose values in blood glucose meters that employ GDH-PQQ chemistry, which led the US Food and Drug Administration (FDA) to issue a public health notification in August 2009[36] to avoid the use of GDH-PQQ glucose test strips being used in many glucose meters.

Mediators

Mediators are an essential component of BGMD to shuttle the electron from the enzyme to the underlying surface of a detecting electrode. The O_2/H_2O_2 redox pair acts as a mediator in GlucoWatch® G2 Biographer (Cygnus, USA), Guardian REAL-Time (Medtronic MiniMed, USA) and DexCom™ STS™-7 (DexCom, Inc., USA) and other BGMD.[37] The detection scheme is based on the FAD-GOx system and uses O_2 as an oxidizing agent (equation 5). The use of dioxygen can lead to a severe limitation known as 'oxygen deficit',[38] i.e. lower O_2 concentration in comparison to the glucose concentration in IF,[39] which introduces variable sensor response and decreases the upper limit of glucose detection. However, a glucose limiting membrane is used in the test strips to obviate this limitation. An alternative mediator can also facilitate the redox reaction between FAD-/FADH$_2$-GOx and M_{red}/M_{ox} (equation 6). It competes with O_2 and reacts rapidly with enzyme cofactors at low redox potential, which obviates the interference from electroactive biomolecules such as uric acid, ascorbic acid, acetaminophen, etc. The most widely used mediators in test strips are ferrocene-derivatives,[40–43] $Os^{2+/3+}$ complexes[44] and ferricyanide.

$$H_2O_2 \rightarrow 2H^+ + O_2 + 2E^- \tag{5}$$
$$FADH_2 - GOx + 2M_{ox} \rightarrow FAD - GOx + 2M_{red} + 2H^+ \tag{6}$$
$$2M_{red} \rightarrow 2M_{ox} + 2e^- \tag{7}$$

The first generation of BGMD employed ferrocene and its derivatives,[46] small molecules that can approach the active site of the enzyme,[47–49] as a mediator for the GOx-based enzymatic reaction.[50–53] An example is the use of 1,1'-dimethyl-3-(2-amino-1-hydroxyethyl)

TABLE 2.2 Characteristics of commercial BGMS. (Reproduced with permission from Elsevier B.V.[45])

Company	Products	Detection method	Enzyme	Sample	Sampling site	Sample size (μL)	Test time (s)	Range (mg dL⁻¹)
Abbott	FreeStyle Navigator®	Amperometric (CGMS), Coulometric (BGMS)	WIRED ENZYME™ technology	Whole blood, capillary	Upper arm, forearm, hand, fingertips, thigh and calf	0.3 (BGMS)	7	20–500
	FreeStyle Freedom® Lite	Coulometric	GDH	Whole blood, capillary	Upper arm, forearm, hand, fingertips, thigh and calf	0.3	5	20–500
	FreeStyle® Lite	Coulometric	GDH	Whole blood, capillary	Upper arm, forearm, hand, fingertips, thigh and calf	0.3	5	20–500
	Precision Xtra™	Amperometric	GDH	Whole blood, capillary	Upper arm, forearm, hand, fingertips, thigh and calf	0.6	5	20–500
	MediSense® Optium™ Xceed™	Amperometric	GDH	Whole blood, capillary	Fingertips, forearm, upper arm, base of the thumb	0.6	5	20–500
Minimed	Guardian®	Amperometric	GOx	Whole blood, capillary	CGMS	Continuous	Real-time	40–400
Dexcom	Seven®	Amperometric	GOx	Whole blood, capillary	CGMS	Continuous	Real-time	40–400

Company	Products	Detection method	Enzyme	Sample	Sampling site	Sample size (µL)	Test time (s)	Range (mg dL⁻¹)
	SEVEN® PLUS	Amperometric	GOx	Whole blood, capillary	CGMS	Continuous	Real-time	40–400
Roche Diagnostics	ACCU-CHEK® Compact Plus	Reflectance photometric	GDH	Whole blood, capillary	Fingertips, palm, forearm, upper arm, thigh, and calf	1.5	5	10–600
	ACCU-CHEK® Active	Reflectance photometric	GDH	Whole blood, capillary	Fingertips	1–2	5	10–600
	ACCU-CHEK® Aviva	Amperometric	GDH	Whole blood, capillary	Fingertips, palm, forearm, upper arm, thigh, and calf	0.6	5	10–600
	ACCU-CHEK® Advantage							
	ACCU-CHEK® Compact							
	ACCU-CHEK® Complete							
Bayer	BREEZE® 2	Amperometric	GOx	Whole blood, capillary	Fingertips, palm, and forearm	1	5	20–600
	Contour®	Amperometric	GDH	Whole blood	Fingertips, palm, and forearm	0.6	5	20–600

Company	Products	Detection method	Enzyme	Sample	Sampling site	Sample size (µL)	Test time (s)	Range (mg dL⁻¹)
	Ascensia Elite™	Amperometric	GOx	Whole blood	Finger, alternative puncture site within certain conditions	2	30	20–600
	Ascensia Elite™ XL	Amperometric	GOx	Whole blood	Finger, alternative puncture site within certain conditions	2	30	20–600
Lifescan	One Touch® Ultra® 2	Amperometric	GOx	Whole blood, capillary	Fingertip, forearm, and palm	1	5	20–600
	One Touch® Ultra Link™	Amperometric	GOx	Whole blood, capillary	Fingertip, forearm, and palm	1	5	20–600
	One Touch® UltraMini™	Amperometric	GOx	Whole blood, capillary	Fingertip, forearm, and palm	1	5	20–600
	One Touch® Select™	Amperometric	GOx	Whole blood, capillary	Fingertip, forearm, and palm	1	5	20–600
	One Touch® UltraSmart®	Amperometric	GOx	Whole blood, capillary	Fingertip, forearm, and palm	1	5	20–600

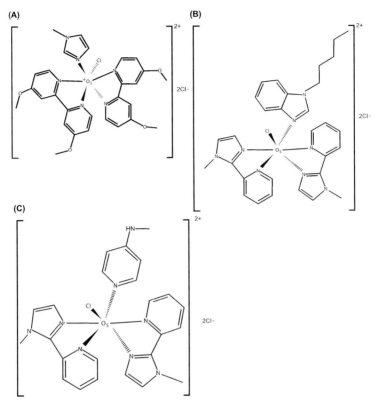

FIGURE 2.2 $Os^{2+/3+}$ complexes used as mediators in the (A) first,[61] (B) second and (C) third generation of Abbott Freestyle test strips.[63] (Reproduced with permission from Elsevier B.V.[45])

ferrocene as a mediator in the MediSense® ExacTech™ and Precision QID™. $Os^{2+/3+}$ complexes are widely employed as mediators for BGMD by Abbott as they transfer electrons rapidly between the redox centres of enzymes and the electrode surface.[54–61] The use of Os polypyridine-based complexes as a mediator in the PQQ-GDH based Abbott Freestyle test strips (Fig. 2.2A)[62] reduces the glucose response time to <15 s at –125 mV vs. Ag/AgCl. However, an improved mediator based on Os polypyridine-based complexes (Fig. 2.2B) further reduces the response time to just 5 s. Subsequently, the shifting of PQQ-GDH-based test strips to FAD-GDH-based strips and further improvement in mediator (Fig. 2.2C) leads to higher current response at –160 mV vs. Ag/AgCl with an assay time of 5 s.

Ferricyanide is a fast mediator for the enzymatic reaction[64–67] in many test strips such as Bayer Contour™ and LifeScan OneTouch® Ultra®. Similarly, nitrosoaniline is used as the precursor of the

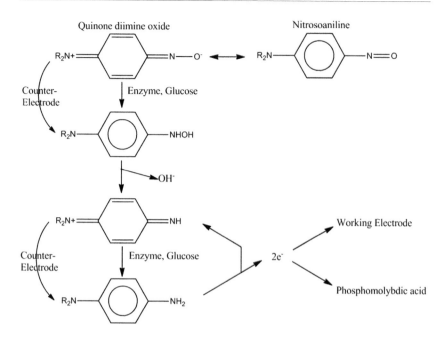

FIGURE 2.3 The mediator system used in Roche glucose sensing test strips.[67] (Reproduced with permission from Elsevier B.V.[45])

mediator in glucose sensing strips of Roche Diagnostics (Fig. 2.3).[68] The mediator is produced by the reaction of nitrosoaniline with an enzyme (e.g. GOx, PQQ- and FAD-GDH) and glucose.

The glucose testing in BGMD can be affected by interference from physiological substances such as acetaminophen, ascorbic acid, bilirubin, cholesterol, dopamine and uric acid. Moreover, it can also be influenced by a broad range of electrochemical and pharmacological substances such as ibuprofen, tetracycline, salicylic acid, ephedrine, L-DOPA, methyl-DOPA, tolbutamide, tolazamide, creatinine, bilirubin, and triglycerides. At low glucose levels, the readings of Accu-Chek Advantage (Roche) and One Touch (Lifescan) are affected by ascorbic acid (30 mg mL⁻¹) while the readings of Accu-Chek Advantage are affected by acetaminophen and dopamine (20 mg mL⁻¹). Similarly, at high glucose levels, dopamine (40 mg mL⁻¹) interferes with the glucose detection by Accu-Chek Advantage, and acetaminophen (20 mg mL⁻¹) affects the glucose reading of Precision G and Precision QID (Abbott). The first generation of mediators (e.g., ferricyanide) significantly interferes with non-specific substances due to minor kinetic barriers.[69] But the subsequent use of the $Os^{2+/3+}$ based redox mediator, employing an applied potential of $-160\,mV$ vs Ag/AgCl, in FreeStyle BGM meter, obviates most of these potential interferences.

However, an ideal next-generation BGMD would be mediatorless and employ low applied potential for glucose detection, which would be useful in obviating the possible interferences due to electroactive metabolites and non-specific substances. It will possibly be based on the direct electron transfer between glucose and the electrodes.

Wired enzyme

The leaching of enzymes is one of the main problems for CGMS, which leads to reduced shelf life and irreproducible results. Wired enzymes obviated this limitation and resulted in highly stabilised leach-proof glucose biosensors. GOx was modified with carbodiimide-activated ferrocene/ferrocenium redox centres that formed phonon-assisted electron tunnelling paths by the formation of ferrocene carboxamides, thereby leading to the transfer of electrons between the electrode surface and the $FAD/FADH_2$ redox centres buried inside GOx.[70] The leach-proof covalent binding of GOx to electron-conducting hydrogels, comprising of Os polypyridine-based redox centres tethered to the cross-linked water-soluble polymer backbones,[37,63] was demonstrated by Heller and co-workers[69-73] using the wired enzyme technique. The active centres of GOx enveloped in redox hydrogel are electrically connected to electrodes irrespective of the spatial orientation of enzymes,[44,74] which leads to 10–100-fold higher current densities due to the connection of multiple GOx layers.[44,74-76] The wired GOx is formed between the vinyl pyridine polymer and the pendant Os complex[75,76] (Fig. 2.4A), and a cross-linker (Fig. 2.4B) connects the GOx via its amine groups to the pyridyl groups of polymer backbone (Fig. 2.4C). As a result, by cross-linking the polymer chains, an insoluble hydrogel is formed on the electrode surface.[77] The GOx wired hydrogels are three-dimensional electrocatalysts[78,79] with a high current density for glucose detection[76] due to the minimised distance between the electrode surface and the $FAD/FADH_2$ redox centres in GOx, which is useful for the miniaturisation of glucose testing electrodes.[80-82] However, they have a high permeability for glucose, gluconolactone, and the electrolytes, as desired for BGM.

The mechanism for wired GOx-based glucose oxidation involves the initial formation of an electrostatic adduct of GOx (polyanion at pH 7.3) with polycationic redox polymer, which is followed by GOx crosslinking and its incorporation into the $Os^{2+/3+}$ complex-based redox polymers[63] in the water-swollen hydrogel. The oxidation of glucose reduces the FAD reaction centres of wired GOx in redox hydrogel

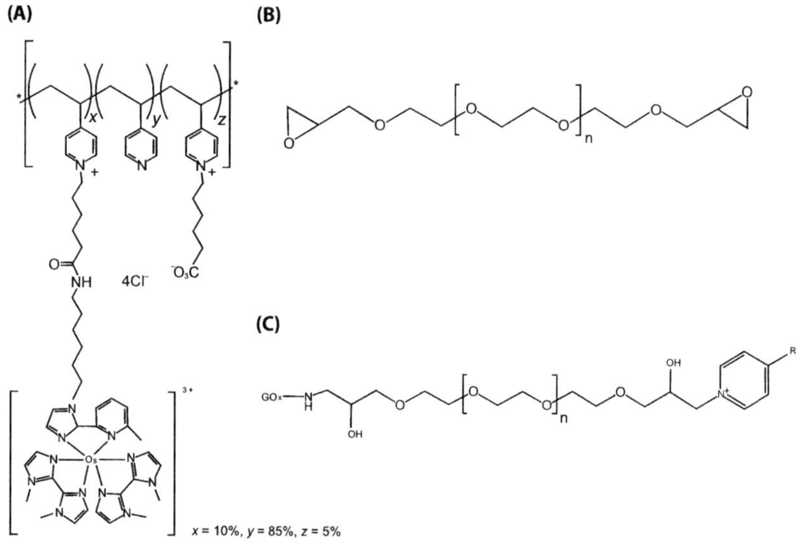

FIGURE 2.4 Chemical structures of (A) redox hydrogels,[75,76] (B) cross-linker, and (C) epoxy linkage for Wired Enzyme™.[68] (Reproduced with permission from Elsevier B.V.[45])

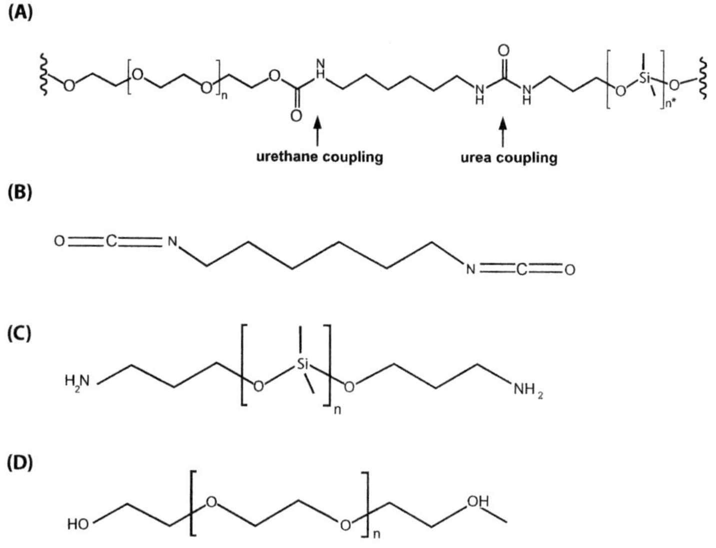

FIGURE 2.5 Chemical structures of (A) polyurethane polyurea block copolymer formed by (B) hexamethylene diisocyanate, (C) aminopropyl-terminated siloxane polymer and (D) polyethylene glycol.[68]

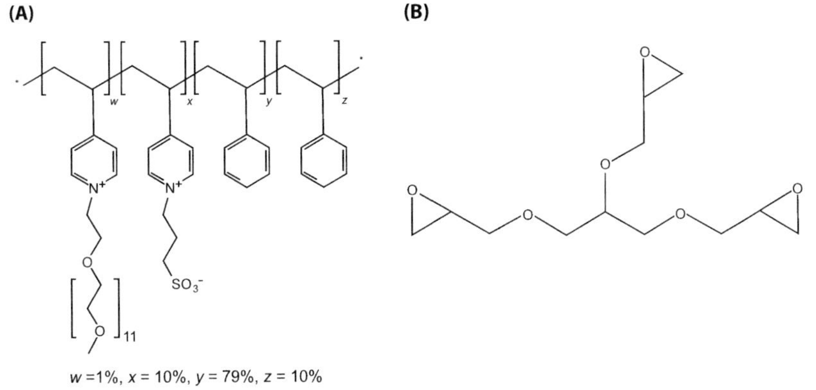

(A)

(B)

$w = 1\%$, $x = 10\%$, $y = 79\%$, $z = 10\%$

FIGURE 2.6 Chemical structures of (A) vinyl pyridine-styrene copolymer and (B) epoxy cross-linker used in FreeStyle Navigator CGMS.[68]

to $FADH_2$, which is followed by its collisions with the Os^{3+} centres and the resulting transfer of electrons/holes. This leads to the reduction of Os^{3+} to Os^{2+} in the hydrogel, which can be re-oxidised back to Os^{3+}. The electron transfer, requiring collisions between reduced and oxidised redox centres,[83,84] is optimum when the hydrogel is poised at its redox potential that has an equal number of reduced and oxidised centres. But it can be enhanced by attaching the redox centres to long and flexible spacers, which enable much better electron transfer due to the increased displacement.[75,76]

Glucose-limiting membrane

A glucose-limiting membrane maximises the availability of O_2 by limiting the excess glucose molecules to react with the enzyme molecules in a BGMD that employs the O_2/H_2O_2 redox pair as a mediator.[85] It enables the detection of higher glucose concentrations by preventing the 'oxygen deficit' and the saturation of the immobilised enzyme at a lower glucose concentration. A vinyl pyridine-styrene copolymer (Fig. 2.6A) with an epoxy cross-linker (Fig. 2.6B) is used as a biocompatible glucose-limiting hydrogel membrane in the FreeStyle Navigator CGMS (Abbott Diabetes Care, CA, USA).[86] In contrast, a polyurethane polymer is used as the glucose-limiting membrane in DexCom™ STS™-7 CGMS (DexCom, Inc., CA, USA) as it reduces the required O_2 concentration, thereby resulting in minimised H_2O_2 production.[87] This is essential for maintaining the functional integrity of CGMS as H_2O_2, being a strong oxidizing substance, that can damage the enzyme activity. Similarly, a proprietary polyurethane polyurea block copolymer, composed of hexamethylene diisocyanate, aminopropyl-terminated siloxane polymer and polyethylene glycol, is used as a glucose-limiting membrane in the Guardian REAL-Time CGMS (Medtronic MiniMed, CA, USA) (Fig. 2.5).[37] As the hydrophobic siloxane and hydrophobic diol are permeable to O_2 and glucose molecules, respectively, the use of an optimum siloxane to diol ratio can obviate the oxygen deficit.

TEST STRIPS

The blood glucose-sensing test strips being used in BGMD are mass produced with very high accuracy and precision. They are cost-effective and have prolonged shelf-life at ambient environmental storage conditions. A usual test strip involves the deposition of the working, counter and reference electrodes onto a plastic substrate. The fill detection electrodes are also used to confirm the automatic filling of blood samples in the test strip, thereby enabling the immediate start of electrochemical glucose sensing assay. A small capillary chamber, coated inside with a dry mixture of enzymes, mediators and other assay components, is positioned on the electrode substrate to work as reaction container. The capillary chamber, having an inlet to receive the blood sample at one end and an outlet to let the displaced air escape at the other end, enables sample uptake of up to 1 mL. The test strips used in the FreeStyle BGMD,[77] the subcutaneous wired GOx electrode[82] and the Freestyle Navigator sensor chip[63] are illustrated in Fig. 2.7.

A working electrode, made from screen-printed carbon ink, vapour-deposited gold or palladium, transmits the electrons derived from the glucose-sensing assay to the glucose meter, which displays the glucose reading of the sample. The required blood sample is kept minimal by minimising the distance between the working and the auxiliary/reference electrode or combining the auxiliary and reference electrodes. The Ag/AgCl electrode is the most commonly used auxiliary/reference electrode that is produced by screen-printing technology using Ag/AgCl ink and polyester as a binding agent. The half-cell reactions are shown by equations (8,9) while the net electrode reaction is shown in equation (10). The simultaneous deposition of the working and auxiliary/reference electrodes onto the substrate also requires an inert auxiliary/reference electrode that is composed of the same material as the working electrode. The working and auxiliary/reference electrodes are assembled in a coplanar or facing electrode configuration, where the facing electrode configuration is preferred as it minimises the distance between the working and the auxiliary/reference

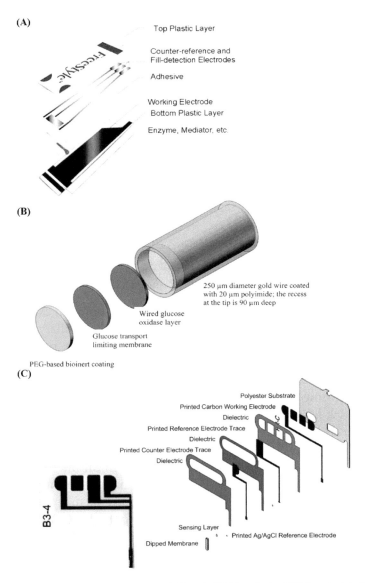

(A)

Top Plastic Layer

Counter-reference and
Fill-detection Electrodes

Adhesive

Working Electrode
Bottom Plastic Layer

Enzyme, Mediator, etc.

(B)

250 μm diameter gold wire coated
with 20 μm polyimide; the recess
at the tip is 90 μm deep

Wired glucose
oxidase layer

Glucose transport
limiting membrane

PEG-based bioinert coating

(C)

Polyester Substrate
Printed Carbon Working Electrode
Dielectric
Printed Reference Electrode Trace
Dielectric
Printed Counter Electrode Trace
Dielectric

B3-4

Sensing Layer
Printed Ag/AgCl Reference Electrode
Dipped Membrane

FIGURE 2.7 The expanded views of Abbott's (A) FreeStyle BGM test strip,[77] (B) subcutaneous wired GOx electrode,[82] and (C) Freestyle Navigator sensor chip.[63]

electrodes, thereby resulting in lower sample requirement and rapid response. But the proximity of these electrodes can induce redox shuttling during glucose oxidation, which shuttles large amounts of mediator back and forth between the electrodes under high potential difference. However, this can be obviated using low applied potential and a rapid enzyme-mediator chemistry, as demonstrated by Abbott FreeStyle BGMD that employs $Os^{2+/3+}$ complex-based chemistry and an applied potential of $-160\,mV$ vs Ag/AgCl, which enables glucose detection in just 5 s.[63]

$$Glucose \rightarrow \delta - Gluconolactone + 2H^+ + 2e^- \text{ (working electrode)} \tag{8}$$

$$AgCl + e^- \rightarrow Ag + Cl^- \tag{9}$$

$$Glucose + 2AgCl \rightarrow \delta - Gluconolactone + 2Ag + 2H^+ \tag{10}$$

As shown in equation 11,[88] the strip filling time of the capillary chamber is directly proportional to the square of chamber length and inversely proportional to capillary thickness and cosine wetting angle. Thus, a rapid BGMD can be developed by decreasing the capillary chamber length and the wetting angle via surfactant treatment.

$$t = \frac{3\mu x^2}{[\delta \cos(\theta_w)]s} \tag{11}$$

where t is filling time, μ is viscosity, x is length along fill axis, δ is liquid surface tension, θ_w is the wetting angle, and s is capillary thickness.

The reagents used in a BGM strip are the enzymes, redox mediators, an enzyme stabiliser, film-forming agents (for glucose limiting, anti-interference, and anti-biofouling membrane) and others such as filling time-reducing surfactants and biocompatible interface. In fingerstick BGM strips, a mixture of enzyme and mediator is usually used to coat the working electrode in aqueous form, which leads to the formation of an active reaction film after evaporation. Sometimes these reagents are initially mixed with the carbon ink and then co-deposited on the substrate. However, this manufacturing method is not suitable for implantable CGMS as the reagents may leach off and dissolve in the subcutaneous fluid. Therefore, the enzyme and the mediator are covalently immobilised in a polymeric membrane in case of CGMS.[88–90]

The most promising advance is the coulometric detection method by Abbott that enables the painless taking off of only 300 nL of a whole blood sample.[78] Abbott's coulometric BGMD has the least sample requirement and improved linearity but same response time and glucose detection range as BGMD from other companies (Table 2.3). However, the reduced sample size from 1 µL to 300 nL has been widely debated and considered non-essential by many as the pricking of the fingertip always provides a few µL of sample.

EMERGING TECHNOLOGIES IN BLOOD GLUCOSE MONITORING

Smartphone-based blood glucose monitoring devices

Smartphones are the ideal POC instruments for personalised healthcare monitoring based on their continuously increasing specifications and features, and successful transfer of many biosensing and bioanalytical applications.[91,92] Other advanced features include the availability of real-time spatiotemporal tagged data, customised text alerts, wireless connectivity, Cloud computing, and telemedicine features including communication and alerts. They have penetrated 98% of the human population (i.e. more than 7 billion subscribers) and more than 70% users live in the developing countries.[93]

The Wireless Smart Gluco-Monitoring System (Fig. 2.8A), developed by iHealth Labs, Inc. (USA), is a cost-effective (US$29.95) smartphone-interfaced electrochemical glucose meter that has been approved by the FDA and Conformité Européenne (CE). The glucose meter determines blood glucose in the range of 1.1–33.3 mmol L^{-1} (mM) using 0.7 µL of fresh capillary whole blood in just 5 s. It has a built-in, rechargeable battery that lasts for up to 200 tests, a light emitting diode (LED) display, and Bluetooth wireless connectivity to the smartphone. It comes with the iHealth Gluco-Smart App, which requires the user to generate a unique iHealth ID that provides access to free and secure iHealth Cloud services where the user can store all

(A)   (B)

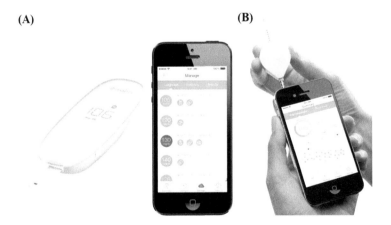

FIGURE 2.8 Smartphone-based glucose meters. (A) Smartphone interfaced iHealth Wireless Smart Gluco-Monitoring System developed by iHealth Inc. (B) iHealth Align, the smallest FDA-approved and CE market smartphone-based glucose meter developed by iHealth Labs, Inc. (Reproduced with permission from iHealth Labs, Inc.)

glucose measurements. The user can see the trends in glycaemic profile and the previous readings of up to 90 days. Moreover, the patient can set up medication alerts and insulin reminders, and can also share readings with family members, friends, and doctors. The smart app also determines the expiration of test strips and analyses the test strips remaining, thereby preventing errors in measurement.

The most recent launch of iOS-enabled iHealth Align, the world's smallest FDA-approved and CE-marked blood glucose meter, is a significant advance in personalised diabetes management. The meter plugs directly into the headphone jack of a smartphone and displays readings of the glucose measurements directly on the smartphone's screen. It is highly cost-effective and can be purchased online at a nominal cost of US$16.95 (Fig. 2.8B).

FreeStyle Libre® flash blood glucose monitoring system

FreeStyle Libre® system is a CGMS launched by Abbott in late 2014, which is approved for sales in Europe. It uses a small sensor patch that measures glucose in just 1 s and performs CGM.[21,22] A coin-sized sensor patch is placed on the back of the upper arm via a simple applicator, followed by scanning of the sensor using a FreeStyle Libre reader® and displaying the glucose measurement reading on the reader's screen (Fig. 2.9). The mobile-sized reader with touchscreen shows the real-time glucose reading, the glucose readings of the previous 8 h and a trend arrow indicating an 'up or down' glucose level. However, the sensor needs to be scanned at least once every 8 h to get all CGM data for a complete glycaemic picture. The scanning works fine even when clothes (1–4 mm thick) are worn. The insertion of the sensor is

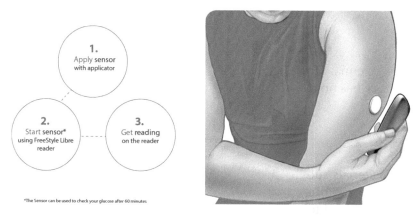

1. Apply sensor with applicator

2. Start sensor* using FreeStyle Libre reader

3. Get reading on the reader

*The Sensor can be used to check your glucose after 60 minutes

FIGURE 2.9 Operation of the FreeStyle Libre® flash blood glucose monitoring system developed by Abbott. (Reproduced with permission from Abbott, USA.)

TABLE 2.3 Comparison of recent commercially available glucose meters. (Reproduced and adapted with permission from Elsevier B.V.[45])

Features	Abbott FreeStyle® Lite	Bayer Contour™ USB	LifeScan OneTouch® Ultra® 2	Roche Diagnostics Accu-Chek® Aviva
CE/FDA Approval	Yes	Yes	Yes	Yes
Enzymes used	GDH	GDH	GOx	GDH
Mediators	Os complex	Ferricyanide	Ferricyanide	Ferricyanide
Enzyme loading	Screen-printing	Screen-printing	Screen-printing	Screen-printing
Sample volume (in µL)	0.3	0.6	1	0.6
Response (in s)	5	5	5	5
Precision (%)	CV≤ 3	CV≤ 5.3	CV≤ 4.4	CV≤2
Haematocrit (%)	15–65	15–65	30–55	20–70
Correlation efficient (γ)	0.98	0.98	0.98	–
Calibration	Plasma Equivalent	Plasma Equivalent	Plasma Equivalent	Plasma Equivalent
Strip needs coding	No	No	Yes	Yes

very simple and its extended life of up to 14 days is a unique feature of the device. The FreeStyle Libre® sensor is factory-calibrated and does not need constant calibration by BGM using test strips. The device is considered as the next generation of glucose monitoring where the need for test strips and lancets has been nearly eliminated except during rapidly changing glucose levels, hypoglycaemia or impending hypoglycaemia. However, as it relies on the scanning of the sensor, the device has no alarm to alert any changes in the glycaemic profile.

Other emerging technologies

Direct electrochemical oxidation is an appealing concept in the work towards the development of a reagentless approach. Various electrode materials such as Au, Pt, Ag, etc. can oxidise glucose but only at extreme alkaline pH. Metal nanoparticles and nanocomposites have been tested to oxidise glucose at neutral pH.[94] However, reproducibility is still problematic, and severe interference by endogenous electroactive molecules (uric acid, ascorbic acid, etc.), novel drugs and their metabolites are highly anticipated. Molecularly imprinted polymers to bio-mimic glucose recognition is another 'enzymeless' approach. As an example, a sensitive layer for glucose can be prepared by electropolymerisation of o-phenylenediamine on a gold electrode in the presence of glucose.[95] To date, no printed polymers have shown the necessary selectivity, detection sensitivity, reproducibility, etc. required for glucose detection.

CONCLUSIONS

BGMD play a prominent role in diabetic monitoring and management as they empower diabetics to maintain their blood glucose levels within the normal physiological range, which will enable them to live a healthy life and obviate life-threatening and costly diabetic complications. The last two decades have witnessed remarkable developments in the field of BGM with many new devices finding their way into the commercial market. There have been considerable improvements in blood glucose sensing chemistries, mediators, glucose-limiting membranes and test strips. This has resulted in the current generation of advanced GMs that have a very fast response, employ miniaturised test strips requiring only a sub-microliter sample, and use minimally invasive, painless lancing of a fingertip. However, unexpected results might come up from time to time and could be attributed to problems with samples or the meter, or user error. The user has to make sure that the test site (fingers) is not contaminated with sugar-based foods, and the patient is not dehydrated or in shock before the test. It is important to avoid squeezing the finger so hard so that blood is not flowing and results in a false low reading. The best test sites are always the patient's clean fingers.

The recent launch of FreeStyle Libre® by Abbott is a breakthrough achievement as it has obviated the need for lancets and test strips. The technology employs a small sensor patch that measures glucose continuously for up to 14 days, stores the glucose readings of up to 8 h, and scans them onto a small reader. However, the current BGM trend is inclined strongly towards smartphone-based devices. The recent launch of iHealth Align's smartphone-based glucose meter is another pioneering advance, which will give diabetics the desired flexibility and freedom to test their blood glucose anywhere at any time, and share and analyse their personalised data securely via a smart app. Further, the long-term vision of developing wearable watch-shaped glucose meters might be a reality very soon following the emergence of smart watch-based healthcare devices and applications. The market for glucose devices has been dominated by giant companies that have made it difficult for start-up counterparts to get involved. Of course, the ultimate goal is the development of biosensors that are fast, accurate and non-invasive, which will mean diabetics are not required to prick their fingers several times every day for the rest of their life.

REFERENCES

1. American Diabetes Association. Standards of medical care in diabetes – 2010. *Diabetes Care*. 2010; 33(Supplement 1): S11–S61.
2. Kolb H, Kempf K, Martin S, Stumvoll M, Landgraf R. On what evidence-base do we recommend self-monitoring of blood glucose? *Diabetes Res Clin Pract*. 2010; 87(2): 150–6.
3. Renard E. Monitoring glycemic control: the importance of self-monitoring of blood glucose. *Am J Med*. 2005; 118(Suppl 9A): 12S–19S.
4. Blonde L, Karter AJ. Current evidence regarding the value of self-monitored blood glucose testing. *Am J Med*. 2005; 118(9): 20–6.
5. Bergenstal RM, Gavin JR, 3rd. Global consensus conference on glucose monitoring. The role of self-monitoring of blood glucose in the care of people with diabetes: report of a global consensus conference. *Am J Med*. 2005; 118(Suppl 9A): 1S–6S.
6. Marks V. Blood glucose: its measurement and clinical importance. *Clin Chim Acta*. 1996; 251(1): 3–17.
7. Newman JD, Warner PJ, Turner APF, Tigwell LJ. *Biosensors: a clearer view*. Cranfield University, UK. 2004: 216.
8. St John A, Davis WA, Price CP, Davis TM. The value of self-monitoring of blood glucose: a review of recent evidence. *J Diabetes Complications*. 2010; 24(2): 129–41.
9. Solnica B, Naskalski JW, Sieradzki J. Analytical performance of glucometers used for routine glucose self-monitoring of diabetic patients. *Clin Chim Acta*. 2003; 331(1–2): 29–35.
10. Girardin CM, Huot C, Gonthier M, Delvin E. Continuous glucose monitoring: a review of biochemical perspectives and clinical use in type 1 diabetes. *Clin Biochem*. 2009; 42(3): 136–42.
11. Lehmann R, Kayrooz S, Greuter H, Spinas GA. Clinical and technical evaluation of a new self-monitoring blood glucose meter: assessment of analytical and user error. *Diabetes Res Clin Pract*. 2001; 53(2): 121–8.
12. Bergenstal RM. Evaluating the accuracy of modern glucose meters. *Insulin*. 2008; 3(1): 5–14.
13. Demir S, Yilmazturk GC, Aslan D. Technical and clinical evaluation of a glucose meter employing amperometric biosensor technology. *Diabetes Res Clin Pract*. 2008; 79(3): 400–4.
14. Kimberly MM, Vesper HW, Caudill SP, Ethridge SF, Archibold E, Porter KH,

et al. Variability among five over-the-counter blood glucose monitors. *Clin Chim Acta*. 2006; 364(1–2): 292–7.

15. Clark LC Jr, Lyons C. Electrode systems for continuous monitoring in cardiovascular surgery. *Annals of the New York Academy of Sciences*. 1962; 102: 29–45.

16. Updike SJ, Hicks GP. The enzyme electrode. *Nature*. 1967; 214(5092): 986–8.

17. Hubert CA. Reflectance meter. United States Patent; 1971; US 3604815A.

18. Kyvik KO, Traulsen J, Reinholdt B, Froland A. The ExacTech blood glucose testing system. *Diabetes Res Clin Pract*. 1990; 10(1): 85–90.

19. Zhang X-E. Screen-printing methods for biosensor production, in J Cooper and T Cass, eds, *Biosensors: a practical approach*. 2nd ed., 2004. Oxford University Press, New York: pp. 41–58.

20. Newman JD, White SF, Tothill IE, Turner AP. Catalytic materials, membranes, and fabrication technologies suitable for the construction of amperometric biosensors. *Anal Chem*. 1995; 67(24): 4594–9.

21. FreeStyle Libre®. https://abbottdiabetescarecouk/our-products/freestyle-libre. 2015.

22. Bailey T, Bode BW, Christiansen MP, Klaff LJ, Alva S. The performance and usability of a factory-calibrated flash glucose monitoring system. *Diabetes Technol Ther*. 2015; 17(11): 787–94.

23. Bai YF, Xu TB, Luong JHT, Cui HF. Direct electron transfer of glucose oxidase-boron doped diamond interface: a new solution for a classical problem. *Anal Chem*. 2014; 86(10): 4910–8.

24. Jany K-D, Ulmer W, Fröschle M, Pfleiderer G. Complete amino acid sequence of glucose dehydrogenase from *Bacillus megaterium*. *FEBS Letters* 1984; 165(1,2): 6–10.

25. Kratzsch PSR, Bunk D, Shao Z, Thym D, Knappe W. Variants of soluble pyrroloquinoline quinone-dependent glucose dehydrogenase. WIPO Patent Publication No. 2002; 2002034919 A1.

26. Oubrie A, Rozeboom HJ, Kalk KH, Olsthoorn AJ, Duine JA, Dijkstra BW. Structure and mechanism of soluble quinoprotein glucose dehydrogenase. *EMBO J*. 1999; 18(19): 5187–94.

27. Duine J, Jzn JF, Van Zeeland J. Glucose dehydrogenase from *Acinetobacter calcoaceticus*: a 'quinoprotein'. *FEBS Letters*. 1979; 108(2): 443–6.

28. Keilin D, Hartree EF. Specificity of glucose oxidase (notatin). *Biochem J*. 1952; 50(3): 331–41.

29. Leskovac V, Trivic S, Wohlfahrt G, Kandrac J, Pericin D. Glucose oxidase from *Aspergillus niger*: the mechanism of action with molecular oxygen, quinones, and one-electron acceptors. *Int J Biochem Cell Biol*. 2005; 37(4): 731–50.

30. Olsthoorn AJ, Duine JA. On the mechanism and specificity of soluble, quinoprotein glucose dehydrogenase in the oxidation of aldose sugars. *Biochem*. 1998; 37(39): 13854–61.

31. Willner I, Baron R, Willner B. Integrated nanoparticle-biomolecule systems for biosensing and bioelectronics. *Biosens Bioelectron*. 2007; 22(9–10): 1841–52.

32. Kulys J, Tetianec L, Ziemys A. Probing *Aspergillus niger* glucose oxidase with pentacyanoferrate (III) aza-and thia-complexes. *J Inorg Biochem*. 2006; 100(10): 1614–22.

33. Sato A, Takagi K, Kano K, Kato N, Duine J, Ikeda T. Ca^{2+} stabilizes the semiquinone radical of pyrroloquinoline quinone. *Biochem J*. 2001; 357: 893–8.

34. Pauly HE, Pfleiderer G. D-glucose dehydrogenase from *Bacillus megaterium* M 1286: purification, properties and structure. *Hoppe-Seyler's Z Physiol Chem*. 1975; 356(10): 1613–23.

35. Tsujimura S, Kojima S, Kano K, Ikeda T, Sato M, Sanada H, et al. Novel FAD-dependent glucose dehydrogenase for a dioxygen-insensitive glucose biosensor. *Biosci Biotechnol Biochem*. 2006; 70(3): 654–9.

36. FDA Public Health Notification: Potentially Fatal Errors with GDH-PQQ Glucose Monitoring Technology. www.fdagov/MedicalDevices/Safety/AlertsandNotices/PublicHealthNotifications/ucm176992htm. 2009.

37. McGarraugh G. The chemistry of commercial continuous glucose monitors. *Diabetes Technol Ther*. 2009; 11 Suppl 1(S1): S17–S24.

38. Wang J. Electrochemical glucose biosensors. *Chem Rev*. 2008; 108(2): 814–25.

39. Ballarin B, Cassani MC, Mazzoni R, Scavetta E, Tonelli D. Enzyme electrodes based on sono-gel containing ferrocenyl compounds. *Biosens Bioelectron*. 2007; 22(7): 1317–22.

40. Laurinavicius V, Razumiene J, Ramanavicius A, Ryabov AD. Wiring of PQQ-dehydrogenases. *Biosens Bioelectron*. 2004; 20(6): 1217–22.

41. Razumiene J, Meškys R, Gureviciene V, Laurinavicius V, Reshetova MD, Ryabov AD. 4-Ferrocenylphenol as an electron transfer mediator in PQQ-dependent alcohol and glucose dehydrogenase-catalyzed reactions. *Electrochem Commun*. 2000; 2(5): 307–11.

42. Antiochia R, Gorton L. Development of a carbon nanotube paste electrode osmium polymer-mediated biosensor for determination of glucose in alcoholic beverages. *Biosens Bioelectron*. 2007; 22(11): 2611–7.

43. Cass AE, Davis G, Francis GD, Hill HA, Aston WJ, Higgins IJ, et al. Ferrocene-mediated enzyme electrode for amperometric determination of glucose. *Anal Chem*. 1984; 56(4): 667–71.

44. Ye L, Haemmerle M, Olsthoorn AJ, Schuhmann W, Schmidt HL, Duine JA, et al. High current density 'wired' quinoprotein glucose dehydrogenase electrode. *Anal Chem*. 1993; 65(3): 238–41.

45. Vashist SK, Zheng D, Al-Rubeaan K, Luong JHT, Sheu FS. Technology behind commercial devices for blood glucose monitoring in diabetes management: a review. *Anal Chim Acta*. 2011; 703(2): 124–36.

46. Alvarez-Icaza M, Kalisz HM, Hecht HJ, Aumann KD, Schomburg D, Schmid

RD. The design of enzyme sensors based on the enzyme structure. *Biosens Bioelectron.* 1995; 10(8): 735–42.

47. Forrow NJ, Sanghera GS, Walters SJ. The influence of structure in the reaction of electrochemically generated ferrocenium derivatives with reduced glucose oxidase. *Journal of the Chemical Society, Dalton Transactions.* 2002(16): 3187–94.

48. Forrow NJ, Walters SJ. Transition metal half-sandwich complexes as redox mediators to glucose oxidase. *Biosens Bioelectron.* 2004; 19(7): 763–70.

49. Viswanathan S, Ho J-A. Dual electrochemical determination of glucose and insulin using enzyme and ferrocene microcapsules. *Biosens Bioelectron.* 2007; 22(6): 1147–53.

50. Shan D, Yao W, Xue H. Electrochemical study of ferrocenemethanol-modified layered double hydroxides composite matrix: application to glucose amperometric biosensor. *Biosens Bioelectron.* 2007; 23(3): 432–7.

51. Qiu J, Peng H, Liang R. Ferrocene-modified Fe_3O_4@SiO_2 magnetic nanoparticles as building blocks for construction of reagentless enzyme-based biosensors. *Electrochem Commun.* 2007; 9(11): 2734–8.

52. Qiu J-D, Deng M-Q, Liang R-P, Xiong M. Ferrocene-modified multiwalled carbon nanotubes as building block for construction of reagentless enzyme-based biosensors. *Sens Actuators B Chem.* 2008; 135(1): 181–7.

53. Qiu JD, Wang R, Liang RP, Xia XH. Electrochemically deposited nanocomposite film of CS-Fc/Au NPs/GOx for glucose biosensor application. *Biosens Bioelectron.* 2009; 24(9): 2920–5.

54. Ohara TJ, Rajagopalan R, Heller A. 'Wired' enzyme electrodes for amperometric determination of glucose or lactate in the presence of interfering substances. *Anal Chem.* 1994; 66(15): 2451–7.

55. Pravda M, Jungar CM, Iwuoha EI, Smyth MR, Vytras K, Ivaska A. Evaluation of amperometric glucose biosensors based on co-immobilisation of glucose oxidase with an osmium redox polymer in electrochemically generated polyphenol films. *Anal Chim Acta.* 1995; 304(2): 127–38.

56. Danilowicz C, Cortón E, Battaglini F. Osmium complexes bearing functional groups: building blocks for integrated chemical systems. *J Electroanal Chem.* 1998; 445(1): 89–94.

57. Reiter S, Habermüller K, Schuhmann W. A reagentless glucose biosensor based on glucose oxidase entrapped into osmium-complex modified polypyrrole films. *Sens Actuators B Chem.* 2001; 79(2): 150–6.

58. Zhang C, Gao Q, Aizawa M. Flow injection analytical system for glucose with screen-printed enzyme biosensor incorporating Os-complex mediator. *Anal Chim Acta.* 2001; 426(1): 33–41.

59. Kurita R, Tabei H, Iwasaki Y, Hayashi K, Sunagawa K, Niwa O. Biocompatible glucose sensor prepared by modifying protein and vinylferrocene monomer composite membrane. *Biosens Bioelectron.* 2004; 20(3): 518–23.

60. Joshi PP, Merchant SA, Wang Y, Schmidtke DW. Amperometric biosensors

based on redox polymer-carbon nanotube-enzyme composites. *Anal Chem.* 2005; 77(10): 3183–8.

61. Scodeller P, Flexer V, Szamocki R, Calvo EJ, Tognalli N, Troiani H, et al. Wired-enzyme core-shell Au nanoparticle biosensor. *J Am Chem Soc.* 2008; 130(38): 12690–7.

62. Taylor C, Kenausis G, Katakis I, Heller A. 'Wiring' of glucose oxidase within a hydrogel made with polyvinyl imidazole complexed with [(Os-4, 4'-dimethoxy-2, 2'-bipyridine) Cl]$^{+/2+1}$. *J Electroanal Chem.* 1995; 396(1): 511–5.

63. Heller A, Feldman B. Electrochemistry in diabetes management. *Acc Chem Res.* 2010; 43(7): 963–73.

64. Okuda J, Wakai J, Sode K. The application of cytochromes as the interface molecule to facilitate the electron transfer for PQQ glucose dehydrogenase employing mediator type glucose sensor. *Anal Lett.* 2002; 35(9): 1465–78.

65. Xiang L, Zhang Z, Yu P, Zhang J, Su L, Ohsaka T, et al. In situ cationic ring-opening polymerization and quaternization reactions to confine ferricyanide onto carbon nanotubes: a general approach to development of integrative nanostructured electrochemical biosensors. *Anal Chem.* 2008; 80(17): 6587–93.

66. Yao H, Hu N. pH-sensitive 'on–off' switching behavior of layer-by-layer films assembled by concanavalin A and dextran toward electroactive probes and its application in bioelectrocatalysis. *J Phys Chem B.* 2009; 113(49): 16021–7.

67. Biscay J, Rama EC, García MBG, Carrazón JMP, García AC. Enzymatic sensor using mediator screen-printed carbon electrodes. *Electroanalysis.* 2011; 23(1): 209–14.

68. Hönes J, Müller P, Surridge N. The technology behind glucose meters: test strips. *Diabetes Technol Ther.* 2008; 10(S1): S10–S26.

69. Degani Y, Heller A. Direct electrical communication between chemically modified enzymes and metal electrodes. I. Electron transfer from glucose oxidase to metal electrodes via electron relays, bound covalently to the enzyme. *J Phys Chem.* 1987; 91(6): 1285–9.

70. Gregg BA, Heller A. Cross-linked redox gels containing glucose oxidase for amperometric biosensor applications. *Anal Chem.* 1990; 62(3): 258–63.

71. Gregg BA, Heller A. Redox polymer films containing enzymes. 1. A redox-conducting epoxy cement: synthesis, characterization, and electrocatalytic oxidation of hydroquinone. *J Phys Chem.* 1991; 95(15): 5970–5.

72. Gregg BA, Heller A. Redox polymer films containing enzymes. 2. Glucose oxidase containing enzyme electrodes. *J Phys Chem.* 1991; 95(15): 5976–80.

73. Degani Y, Heller A. Electrical communication between redox centers of glucose oxidase and electrodes via electrostatically and covalently bound redox polymers. *J Am Chem Soc.* 1989; 111(6): 2357–8.

74. Mano N, Mao F, Heller A. Electro-oxidation of glucose at an increased current density at a reducing potential. *Chem Commun.* 2004(18): 2116–7.

75. Mao F, Mano N, Heller A. Long tethers binding redox centers to polymer backbones enhance electron transport in enzyme 'wiring' hydrogels. *J Am Chem Soc*. 2003; 125(16): 4951–7.

76. Mano N, Mao F, Heller A. On the parameters affecting the characteristics of the 'wired' glucose oxidase anode. *J Electroanal Chem*. 2005; 574(2): 347–57.

77. Feldman B, Brazg R, Schwartz S, Weinstein R. A continuous glucose sensor based on Wired Enzyme™ technology: results from a 3-day trial in patients with type 1 diabetes. *Diabetes Technol Ther*. 2003; 5(5): 769–79.

78. Heller A. Electrical connection of enzyme redox centers to electrodes. *J Phys Chem*. 1992; 96(9): 3579–87.

79. Heller A. Electron-conducting redox hydrogels: design, characteristics and synthesis. *Curr Opin Chem Biol*. 2006; 10(6): 664–72.

80. Pishko MV, Michael AC, Heller A. Amperometric glucose microelectrodes prepared through immobilization of glucose oxidase in redox hydrogels. *Anal Chem*. 1991; 63(20): 2268–72.

81. Csoeregi E, Quinn CP, Schmidtke DW, Lindquist S-E, Pishko MV, Ye L, et al. Design, characterization, and one-point in vivo calibration of a subcutaneously implanted glucose electrode. *Anal Chem*. 1994; 66(19): 3131–8.

82. Csoeregi E, Schmidtke DW, Heller A. Design and optimization of a selective subcutaneously implantable glucose electrode based on 'wired' glucose oxidase. *Anal Chem*. 1995; 67(7): 1240–4.

83. Aoki A, Rajagopalan R, Heller A. Effect of quaternization on electron diffusion coefficients for redox hydrogels based on poly(4-vinylpyridine). *J Phys Chem*. 1995; 99(14): 5102–10.

84. Aoki A, Heller A. Electron diffusion coefficients in hydrogels formed of cross-linked redox polymers. *J Phys Chem*. 1993; 97(42): 11014–9.

85. Van Antwerp WP. Polyurethane/polyurea compositions containing silicone for biosensor membranes. WIPO Patent Publication; 1999; WO1996030431 A1.

86. Mao F, Cho H. Biosensor membranes composed of polymers containing heterocyclic nitrogens. United States Patent; 2005; US8380274 B2.

87. Tapsak MA, Rhodes RK, Shults MC, McClure JD. Techniques to improve polyurethane membranes for implantable glucose sensors. United States Patent; 2007; US7226978 B2.

88. Heller A. Implanted electrochemical glucose sensors for the management of diabetes. *Annu Rev Biomed Eng*. 1999; 1(1): 153–75.

89. Hovorka R. Continuous glucose monitoring and closed-loop systems. *Diabet Med*. 2006; 23(1): 1–12.

90. Klonoff DC. A review of continuous glucose monitoring technology. *Diabetes Technol Ther*. 2005; 7(5): 770–5.

91. Vashist SK, Mudanyali O, Schneider EM, Zengerle R, Ozcan A. Cellphone-based devices for bioanalytical sciences. *Anal Bioanal Chem*. 2014; 406(14): 3263–77.

92. Vashist SK, Luppa PB, Yeo LY, Ozcan A, Luong JHT. Emerging technologies for next-generation point-of-care testing. *Trends Biotechnol.* 2015; 33(11): 692–705.
93. Measuring the Information Society Report. www.ituint/en/ITU-D/Statistics/Pages/publications/mis2015aspx. 2015.
94. Cui H-F, Ye J-S, Zhang W-D, Li C-M, Luong JHT, Sheu F-S. Selective and sensitive electrochemical detection of glucose in neutral solution using platinum–lead alloy nanoparticle/carbon nanotube nanocomposites. *Anal Chim Acta.* 2007; 594(2): 175–83.
95. Cheng Z, Wang E, Yang X. Capacitive detection of glucose using molecularly imprinted polymers. *Biosens Bioelectron.* 2001; 16(3): 179–85.

CHAPTER 3

Non-invasive analytics for point-of-care testing of glucose

Sandeep Kumar Vashist and John HT Luong

CHAPTER SUMMARY

Non-invasive (NI) analytics forms an essential part of diabetic health-care monitoring and management, as reflected by the wide range of commercial personalised devices for point-of-care testing (POCT) currently available on the market. Besides blood glucose, a wide variety of other physiological parameters, such as blood pressure, weight, body analysis, pulse rate, electrocardiography (ECG), blood glucose saturation, sleeping, and physical activity are standard measurements carried out in personalised diabetic healthcare management. Nevertheless, NI glucose monitoring (NGM) has always been the most widely investigated area in POCT that can critically improve diabetic care. An emerging trend is the development of personalised POCT devices using a smartphone (SP)-based NI analytics and wearable technologies. However, the successful implementation of NGM and management lies in overcoming the formidable but not insurmountable technical issues to improve the reliability and calibration of NI instruments. Additionally, robust validation is needed to establish the results obtained under different physiological conditions associated with metabolism, bodily fluid circulation, and blood components. NI measurement must be as precise and reliable as measuring glucose in blood and subject to regulatory approval.

Keywords: non-invasive; analytics; point-of-care testing; glucose; health-care; mobile healthcare.

CONTENTS

INTRODUCTION

Commercial POCT devices have emerged to analyse a broad range of physiological health parameters from cardiac function to clinically relevant analytes, the analysis of breath, skin and eye conditions and other applications. Non-invasive (NI) analytics plays a critical role in healthcare monitoring and management. In particular, diabetic glucose monitoring is always the primary target for any NI analytical technique (NIAT) given its rapidly increasing prevalence and the severe implications associated with the disease, especially when complications arise. In 2010 alone, diabetes exacted an annual economic toll of US$376 billion,[1] accounting for a significant proportion of healthcare resources. In 2013, the number of diabetics (366 million) had already surpassed the initial projected number of diabetics for 2030 by the World Health Organization (WHO),[2] which subsequently issued a global wake-up call to plan and implement strategies to counteract this foremost healthcare concern. According to the International Diabetes Federation, it is estimated that the 415 million diabetics at present will rise to 642 million by 2040.[3]

While current finger prick tests provide a more accurate determination of blood glucose levels compared to blood from other less sensitive areas, these tests are still painful, especially for young children, due to the high concentration of sensory nerve endings at the fingertips. This has led to poor patient compliance, wherein a large proportion of diabetic patients only test their blood glucose once or twice a day, which is well below the daily recommendation of 4–7 times. The development of prospective NI glucose monitoring, a viable non-invasive or painless technique, has received considerable attention over the last two decades. The development of a clinically accurate NGM device will be a breakthrough in diabetic monitoring as it can alleviate the pain of finger pricking and the requirement of consumable test strips. Moreover, it will provide the technology for more frequent monitoring of glucose that will lead to increased adherence by end-users. A large number of non-invasive analytical techniques (NIATs), such as Raman spectroscopy, reverse iontophoresis, ultrasound, infrared spectroscopy, polarimetry, photoacoustic spectroscopy, thermal emission spectroscopy and other techniques, have been employed for NGM.[4] Several commercially viable prototypes, such as GlucoWatch® G2 biographer, Pendra®, OrSense NBM-200G, Symphony® and GlucoTrack™, have also been developed.

A recent trend is the development of wearable and smartphone-based technologies[5,6] for personalised mobile healthcare (mH). These devices target parameters such as blood pressure, weight, body analysis, pulse rate, electrocardiograph (ECG), blood glucose, blood glucose saturation, sleeping, and physical activity.[7] In the last few years, several personalised mH devices have been commercialised. It is expected that advances in these wearable and smartphone-based technologies will lead to the development of personalised mH management of diabetes. This chapter focuses on non-invasive POCT of glucose, and the associated current state of the art, technical challenges, and future trends.

NON-INVASIVE ANALYTICAL TECHNIQUES AND THEIR APPLICATIONS

NGM is broadly classified into subcutaneous, dermal, epidermal and combined dermal, and epidermal glucose measurements, although subcutaneous measurement is not strictly an NI technique considering it includes microdialysis, wick extraction, and implanted electrochemical or competitive fluorescence sensors. NI optical measurement is very appealing as it is just performed by focusing a light beam onto a target site on the body. The diffused light represents an optical signature or fingerprint of the tissue content in the sensing area. However, the resulting spectrum is governed by the chemical composition and distribution of the primary chemicals in the tissue matrix as well as the temperature and pressure of living tissue. Therefore, it is challenging to extract glucose-specific quantitative information from the obtained spectrum, given that the signal is often overwhelmed by much larger sources of spectral variance.

Infrared spectroscopy

The skin has two principal layers: the outermost layer known as the epidermis and a second layer called the dermis, which are composed mainly of collagen, elastin and blood capillaries. Although the dermis is the targeted region for optical analysis, glucose molecules are most present in the interstitial fluid (IF) at the epidermis–dermis interface.[8] This fluid provides an additional source of glucose for cells, and its glucose level is proportional to that in the blood but with a delay of about 10 min. In other words, a glucose level reading from IF will correspond to the blood sugar level 10 min prior.

IR measurement systems at the epidermal surface have a penetration depth of 10–50 μm. Its direct measurement of glucose in the blood is both pH and temperature dependent and subject to interference from red blood cells, albumin, and γ-globulin. In addition, salivary glucose can be contaminated with food glucose, leading to considerable variation in the blood glucose levels, thereby rendering it a poor technique. Near-infrared (NIR) and mid-infrared (MIR) spectroscopy are the most commonly used NIATs for glucose monitoring in the ear lobe, finger web, finger cuticle, forearm, lip mucosa and other sites. NIR spectroscopy involves an incident light beam with a wavelength of 750–2500 nm[9-13] on the body's target site to quantify the glucose concentration in tissues (1–100 mm deep) by measuring the changes in the light intensity due to transmission and reflectance in the tissue. However, the absorption coefficient of glucose in the NIR band is much lower than that of water due to the large difference in their concentrations, which causes the overlapping of weak spectral bands of glucose by the stronger NIR spectra of water, haemoglobin (Hb), proteins, and fats. Moreover, NIR measurements are affected by changes in body temperature, blood pressure, skin hydration, skin thickness and skin thermal properties,[14-16] disease states such as hyperglycemia and hyperinsulinemia,[17-19] and concentrations of triglyceride and albumin. Additionally, they are affected by environmental variations, for example, that in temperature, humidity, atmospheric pressure and carbon dioxide content. As such, most NIR-based NGM measurements lack the desired clinical accuracy.

An example is the OrSense NBM-200G, a CE approved portable device which facilitates NI measurement of glucose, Hb, and oxygen saturation. It employs red-NIR occlusion spectroscopy[20] that involves temporary cessation of the blood flow at the fingertip using projected light at 610 nm and 810 nm, which enhances the red-NIR signal, thereby improving the signal-to-noise ratio (SNR). The device measures glucose within a minute, stores up to 500 readings, and is equipped with other desired features such as an easy-to-read display, alarm alerts, trend data analysis and wireless telemetry. It enables continuous glucose monitoring (CGM) for a day without requiring frequent calibration, and is safe for use by patients without any risk of contamination. The device's precision, obtained from over 400 subjects, is comparable to that of blood glucose meters. Additionally, the NGM data enables the identification of glucose trends and the detection of hypo- and hyperglycaemia events. A clinical trial, conducted at the Sheba Medical Center, Israel, shows 95.3%, 4.7% and 0% measurements in the A+B, C+D and E zones of the Clarke error grid analysis (EGA), respectively. SugarTrack (USA, using 650 nm, 880 nm, 940 nm and 1300 nm) and Sensys (USA, using 750–2500 nm) are other NIR-based NGM devices. Of note is a portable NGM detector that detects blood glucose in the capillaries of a finger in one second.[21] Table 3.1 provides a description of prospective NIAT-based NGM devices that have been developed to date.

MIR spectroscopy is based on the same principle as that of NIR spectroscopy except that it employs light with a wavelength of 2500–10000 nm[22–26] to reduce scattering and improve absorption in comparison to NIR, thereby resulting in sharper glucose spectral bands. However, it has the same limitations as NIR in addition to poorer penetration of light into the skin, i.e. only a few micrometres.[27] An advance in this technique is the development of quantum cascade lasers that are capable of producing one of a number of frequencies by passing electrons through a 'cascade' of semiconductor layers for MIR applications.[28] However, it is still a formidable task to shrink this type of laser for portable consumer use, especially if it is to be operated at room temperature without a cooling system.

Attenuated total reflection (ATR), using a light beam guided through a crystal by total reflection, has been employed to increase the penetration of light,[27] wherein the glucose measurement is carried out by placing the crystal in contact with the skin using squalane oil.[29] It measures the glucose concentration in the IF in the dermis from the

TABLE 3.1 Non-invasive analytical technology (NIAT)-based glucose monitoring devices

Device	Company	NIAT employed	Target site	Approval(s)
GlucoWatch© G2 Biographer	Animas Technologies (Cygnus Inc.)	Reverse iontophoresis	Wrist skin	CE, FDA
Pendra©	Biovotion AG (Solianis Monitoring AG; Pendragon)	Bioimpedance spectroscopy	Wrist skin	CE
GlucoTrack™	Integrity Applications Ltd	Ultrasound, electromagnetic and heat capacity	Ear lobe skin	N.M.*
OrSense NBM-200G	OrSense Ltd	Occlusion NIR spectroscopy	Fingertip skin	CE
N.M.*	SpectRx Inc. (Guided Therapeutics, Inc.)	Laser microporation	Skin	N.M.*
Symphony™	Echo Therapeutics, Inc. (Sontra Medical Corporation)	Prelude® SkinPrep System	Skin	N.M.*
HG1-c	C8 Medisensors	Raman spectroscopy	Skin	CE

* Not mentioned

electromagnetic field created by the reflected light.[30] However, these MIR-based glucose measurements, usually conducted on the finger skin or oral mucosa,[31] are affected by the skin's water content.[27]

Reverse iontophoresis

Reverse iontophoresis[32] is based on the transport of glucose out of the skin in the direction opposite to that of iontophoresis, which is used extensively to deliver drugs through the skin by applying an electrical current. An electric potential is applied between an anode and a cathode positioned on the skin surface, which causes the Na^+ and Cl^- ions from beneath the skin to migrate towards the cathode and anode, respectively,[33] thereby generating the electric current.[34] The uncharged glucose molecules in the IF are carried along with the ions across the skin and collected at the cathode, where the glucose concentration is determined by a conventional glucose sensor. This

TABLE 3.2 Advantages and disadvantages of different non-invasive glucose measurement techniques

Measurement procedures	Advantages	Disadvantages
Infrared and Near infrared (NIR)	High sensitivity, less expensive than MIR. Mature technology and availability (hardware and software).	Scanning pressure is applied. Physiological parameter differences not related to blood glucose. Hardware stability.
Midinfrared (MIR)	Low scattering. Sharper glucose peak compared to that of NIR.	Still poor penetration (a few microns). Interference from the water.
Reverse iontophoresis	The electrodes are easily applied to the skin. More reliable measurement (high correlation between the glucose level in a physiological fluid and blood).	Skin irritation. Lengthy deployment time (60 min). Sensitive to sweat and not applicable for detecting rapid changes in blood glucose.
Bioimpedance	Easy to use, inexpensive and does not require complicated population-specific prediction models.	Temperature and water effect remains problematic. Long wait times (60 min).
Raman	Sharper and less overlapped spectra compared to NIR. Less sensitive to temperature variations and the signal associated with water.	Long acquisition times associated with instability of the laser wavelength and intensity. Must be performed at low energy to prevent injury, i.e. a very low signal-to-noise ratio. Interference from other compounds.
Fluorescence	Very sensitive, minimal damage to the body. Measurement of fluorescence intensity and decay times independent of light scattering and fluorophore concentration.	Strong scattering. Short lifetimes and biocompatibility of the fluorescent donor or acceptor.
Optical polarimetry	Visible light and miniaturised optical components.	Poor selectivity for glucose. Sensitive to the scattering properties of tissue. Sensitivity in the reading due to eye movement and motion.

(*continued*)

Measurement procedures	Advantages	Disadvantages
Ultrasound	Higher sensitivity than other spectroscopy techniques.	Sensitive to some biological compounds, temperature/pressure fluctuations, and other environmental parameters. Subject to scattering phenomena (similar to NIR). Expensive.
Electromagnetic	Safe, no ionisation of tissue. Measurement can be specific for glucose at a given frequency range.	Highly dependent on temperature and other blood components other than glucose.
Optical coherence tomography	High resolution and high signal to noise ratio. High penetration depth.	Highly sensitive to motion and temperature.

NIAT has been used in several NGM devices. However, it has several limitations, such as the interference of glucose measurements with sweat from the subject, the duration needed for sufficient glucose to be collected for analysis, and skin irritation.

An example is the GlucoWatch® G2 Biographer (Cygnus Inc., California, USA), a wristwatch-shaped NGM device that received CE certification and FDA approval in 1999 and 2001, respectively. It was approved as an adjunct to blood glucose meters to detect glucose level trends and track patterns in diabetics. The IF was extracted from the skin by reverse iontophoresis[35] by applying a 300 μA electric current between the two electrodes contacting the skin on the rear side of the device. An amperometric biosensor then detects the glucose concentration from the amount of H_2O_2 generated by the common glucose oxidase catalysed reaction.[36] The skin temperature and perspiration fluctuations in subjects are taken into account by employing thermal transducers and conductivity sensors.[37] The device detects glucose with a 15 min time lag compared to the standard glucose meter, requires a 2–3 h warm-up period[38,39] and can perform six glucose measurements per hour. It is equipped with additional general device features for diabetic monitoring, such as alarms for greater deviation in glucose levels, a trend indicator, event markers, data download, software analysis and data storage. Nevertheless, it requires calibration with a glucose meter, a warm-up period before the measurement, and replacement of the disposable pad every 12 h. Moreover, it is not water-resistant and leads to inaccurate measurements if the patient is moving, exercising, sweating or has rapid temperature changes. Additionally, it causes skin irritation and shuts down in the case of sweating, which is also a symptom of hypoglycaemia when NGM is highly desired. Further, it is three times more expensive than the glucose meter. Clinical studies have shown that it performs adequately at high glucose levels but is unreliable in hypoglycaemia.[39] Cygnus Inc. folded in 2004 and was sold to Animas Corporation and Animas Technologies LLC in 2005 followed by the termination of GlucoWatch® G2 Biographer's sales in 2007.

Another NGM device based on the similar concept of laser microporation was developed by SpectRx Inc. (Norcross, Georgia, USA). It employs a handheld Altea MicroPor™ laser to create micropores in the stratum corneum (the outermost layer of skin), which enables the IF to permeate out such that it can be collected using an external patch on the skin for measurement of the glucose concentration with a sensor. The results of the analysis can then be transmitted wirelessly to a handheld display. The device detects 60–400 mg/dL of glucose in the IF but requires calibration with a glucose meter. The results correlate well with those from the clinical analyser and glucose meter, which led to the licensing of the technology to Abbott Laboratories. The name of the corporation changed to Guided Therapeutics, Inc. in 2008 with a shift in the major focus towards the NI detection of cervical precancer and cancer. The company developed the LuViva® advanced cervical scan NIAT, which differentiates between diseased and healthy tissue by analysing light reflected from the cervix.

Similarly, Symphony® was another continuous NGM device developed by Sontra Medical Corporation, which merged with Echo Therapeutics, Inc., a specialty transdermal therapeutics company, in 2007. This NIAT involves the permeation of the skin by a unique transdermal permeation system known as Prelude® SkinPrep. After a brief warm-up period, measurement of glucose every minute on the permeated site follows using a glucose biosensor, with the data wireless transmitted to a remote monitor that is equipped with alarm alerts if the glucose level exceeds the normal range. The device demonstrated adequate performance in the clinical trials conducted in 2011 without causing skin irritation with the results agreeing well with those obtained by the YSI 2300 STAT Plus analyser and glucose meter.

Bioimpedance spectroscopy

The technique involves the measurement of the impedance (dielectric) spectrum of tissue at different wavelengths in the frequency range of 100 Hz–100 MHz using alternating currents of known intensity. The changes in the plasma glucose concentration lead to changes in the Na$^+$ and K$^+$ ion concentrations, thereby resulting in an altered membrane potential of red blood cells (RBCs),[41] which is determined by measurement of the impedance spectrum.[42,43] However, this NIAT is affected by the water content and the disease states affecting the cell membrane. The technique was used in Pendra® (Fig. 3.1A), a wristwatch-shaped NGM device from Pendragon Medical Ltd, Switzerland, which was CE approved in 2003 as an adjunct to glucose meters to detect trends and patterns in glucose levels. An open resonant circuit (1–200 MHz) is in contact with skin via a tape on the rear side of the device and performs up to four impedance measurements per minute with sensitivity in the range of 20–60 mg/dL glucose per Ohm. While Pendra® incorporates all the desired routine features

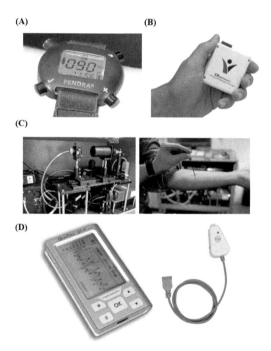

FIGURE 3.1 Non-invasive analytical technology-based devices. (A) Pendra® NGM device. (B) HG1-c continuous NGM device developed by C8 Medisensors. (C) (left) Raman spectroscopy-based NGM device prototype developed by a group of researchers at Massachusetts Institute of Technology, and (right) its use for NGM in interstitial fluid. (D) GlucoTrack™ NGM device: (left) main unit and (right) personal ear clip. (A) Reproduced with permission from Springer International Publishing AG.[40] (B–D) Reproduced with permission from Elsevier B.V.[4]

for diabetic monitoring and management apart from integral self-correction for varying impedance due to changes in temperature, it requires additional personalised calibration to take into account differences in skin and underlying tissues among individuals. Moreover, it was found that about 30% of patients could not use Pendra® following calibration as their skin types, and basic skin impedances, are unsuitable for the device: the device can only be used for a specific cohort whose local skin dielectric possessed a minimum resonance frequency.[44] Further, the Pendra® tape needs to be changed every 24 h and the device reattached at the same spot where it was calibrated. This is followed by a 1 h equilibration period during which the patient must rest before the glucose measurements can be made.[45] The studies show a weak correlation of only 35.1% with regard to glucose meters, while the Clarke EGA indicated 78.4%, 6.5%, 10.8% and 4.3% in the readings in the A+B, C, D and E zones, respectively.[46] The mean absolute difference in comparison with capillary blood glucose values is only 52%. Notwithstanding the bankruptcy of Pendragon Medical Ltd in 2005 at which production of Pendra® was discontinued, bioimpedance spectroscopy remains simple and easy to use; that is, it is a technique that does not require sophisticated and population-specific prediction models.

Raman spectroscopy

Raman spectroscopy employs a visible to MIR range laser radiation source to measure scattered light, which has higher wavelength and lower intensity than the incident light, in transparent samples.[47] This NIAT has the advantage that water does not interfere with the specific Raman spectra for glucose due to its weak scattering index. Moreover, the Raman spectra are narrow with distinct peaks, which makes it simple to separate the desired glucose signals.[47] However, the extended spectral acquisition times and the instability of the laser intensity and wavelength are potential limitations. Glucose detection sensitivity can be improved and the spectral acquisition time decreased by employing surface-enhanced Raman spectroscopy. A compact and water-resistant continuous NGM device, i.e. HG1-c (Fig. 3.1B), was developed by C8 MediSensors (San Jose, California, USA). The CE approved device measures glucose in 3 min with a claimed accuracy comparable to that of the continuous glucose monitoring systems. Moreover, it is highly cost-effective as the cost of continuous glucose determination is less than that of three finger prick tests per day over 4 years. Despite raising a substantial investment funding of US$24 million in 2012, the investment by GE Healthcare through its healthy imagination fund and the scheduled product launch in Europe, C8 MediSensors ceased to function in 2012 due to unknown reasons. Elsewhere, researchers at Massachusetts Institute of Technology demonstrated a miniaturised laptop-sized Raman-based device[48] (Fig. 3.1C) that measures glucose levels in IF by shining the finger or arm with NIR light that penetrates only 0.5 mm below the skin. An algorithm to determine the blood glucose level of the glucose concentration in IF was also developed along with a dynamic concentration correction-based calibration procedure, which improves the accuracy of glucose measurements by taking into account the rate of glucose diffusion from the blood into the IF.[48]

For an optimal collection of glucose-specific Raman-scattered photons and calibration transfer, the probing depth and sample positioning must be well defined. Accordingly, several technical issues must be overcome to enhance glucose specificity and to correct for diversity across individuals. Besides a robust site interface and optimal site determination, the fluorescence background must be significantly suppressed. The interstitial glucose lags the plasma glucose concentration by 4 to 10 min in humans,[49] and thus methods of extracting IF for reference glucose measurements need to be developed. Another considerable drawback is the instability in the laser wavelength/intensity and lengthy spectral acquisition times.

Photoacoustic and ocular spectroscopy

Photoacoustic spectroscopy involves the interaction arising from a laser beam projected onto tissue cells, in which heat is generated, giving rise to acoustic signals in the sample that can be monitored by a piezoelectric transducer.[31] Blood glucose can be detected selectively using an incident laser beam of a specific wavelength.[50] This NIAT can use a laser light with a wide wavelength range from ultraviolet (UV) to NIR, and is unaffected by the water content of skin due to its poor photoacoustic response. Potential limitations include its sensitivity to changes in temperature, pressure and other ambient parameters, and interferences from physiological substances. An NGM device from Glucon (USA), Aprise, was demonstrated to have good correlation with blood glucose levels but possessed potential concerns from reduced sensitivity and non-specific interference from physiological substances. Nevertheless, the device showed an excellent correlation between the photoacoustic signals obtained from the index fingers of healthy and diabetic patients and their blood glucose levels.

Ocular spectroscopy is another prospective NIAT that measures glucose concentration in tears, using a 7-µm-thick boronic acid derivatives-based hydrogel wafer bound onto a contact lens, based on the formation of reversible covalent bonds by the boronic acid derivatives with glucose in tears.[51] The procedure involves the illumination of the contact lens by a light source and the monitoring of the change in wavelength of reflected light due to the glucose concentration in tears by a spectrometer. Limitations include the discomfort of using contact lenses, the difference in results from both eyes, and problems with calibration, such as in persons with poor eyesight. Other shortcomings are the reproducibility in obtaining the desired tear sample, the time lag between the glucose concentration in blood and tears, and the poor correlation between blood and tear glucose.[52] Moreover, this approach requires significant improvements regarding increased biocompatibility, lifetime and signal resolution.

Polarimetry and fluorescence

Polarimetry is based on passing polarised light through a solution containing optically active solutes such as glucose, which causes the rotation of the linear polarisation vector of light depending on the thickness, temperature and analyte concentration in the sample. Although the change in the optical signal by glucose is small, glucose is a good optical rotator. Skin is inappropriate for such NIATs due to its high scattering coefficients that cause the complete depolarisation of light. The aqueous humour in the anterior chamber of the human eye is ideal for such NGM as it constitutes clear optical media with an appropriate path length.[53,54] The polarimetric tests in the eye have two optical paths: where the incident beam passes laterally through the cornea;[54] and where the incident beam on the cornea travelling into the eyeball gets reflected by the retina and returns with information about the glucose concentration in the aqueous humour.[55] The technique has the advantage that it is unaffected by changes in temperature and pH. Nevertheless, significant limitations arise due to the optical noise associated with non-specific substances, safety concerns for the exposure of the eye to light, the need for technology to measure small angles, and the effect of the scattering of light by the tissues on the glucose measurements. Moreover, there is a time lag in the glucose concentration of aqueous humour from that of blood glucose in addition to the poor specificity of glucose measurements in physiological fluids due to interference with several optically active solutes. *In vivo* glucose measurements were also performed on the human eye using a modified intraocular lens and a liquid-crystal polarisation modulator driven by a sinusoidal signal.[56,57]

Another NIAT employs fluorescence-based detection that involves the excitation of tissues by UV light at specific frequencies followed by its detection at a particular wavelength. It was employed for the detection of glucose in tears by using polymerised crystalline colloidal arrays that diffract visible light in response to glucose concentrations.[22] However, ongoing efforts are dedicated to developing contact lenses that can change colour in response to varying glucose concentrations, thereby obviating the need for excitation and detection devices.[58] A prospective study involved the use of UV laser light to excite the glucose solution and to measure the resulting fluorescence signal at 380 nm.[59] The signal was unaffected by fluctuations in the ambient light intensity but is dependent on epidermal thickness, skin pigmentation and other parameters.[53] Apart from the use of UV laser light in tissues that will have high scattering, this NIAT has the same limitations as ocular spectroscopy.[60,61]

Ultrasound, thermal emission spectroscopy, and electromagnetic sensing

Ultrasound-based NIAT is based on the creation of 20 kHz ultrasound using a piezoelectric transducer, which transports glucose to the epidermis by increasing the permittivity of skin to the IF, from which the glucose concentration can be determined using an electrochemical sensor.[54] Thermal emission spectroscopy is based on the measurement of naturally emitted IR signals generated in the human body due to the glucose concentration, which has absorptive effects on the IR radiation directly proportional to its concentration. The glucose detection can be carried out on the forearm, fingertip or ear lobe at specific wavelengths for glucose, i.e. 9.8 μm and 10.9 μm.[21] However, the preferred site is the tympanic membrane as the IR signals pertinent to glucose detection in the blood vessels have to traverse smaller path lengths. This NIAT has high reproducibility[59] but is prone to potential interferences from temperature, body movements and various pathophysiological factors that induce variations in temperature.[60] The electromagnetic sensing-based NIAT is based on the change in dielectric parameters of the blood in response to varying glucose concentration, which can be detected using electromagnetic sensors based on eddy currents.[61,62] Electromagnetic waves at specific frequencies can be used to detect blood glucose, although the skin reflects most of these waves. Localised nuclear magnetic resonance has also been demonstrated for the detection of glycogen metabolism in the human brain,[63] although the measurements are strongly affected by temperature variations and physiological changes in the dielectric parameters of blood.

A prospective handheld NGM device, GlucoTrack™ (Fig. 3.1D),

developed by Integrity Applications Ltd (Ashkelon, Israel), employs three NIATs based on ultrasonic, electromagnetic sensing and heat capacity measurements.[64] This combinatorial approach decreases the noise by minimising the effect of interferences, thereby providing high precision and accuracy. A personal ear clip equipped with sensors and calibration electronics measures the glucose concentration in the ear lobe. The device requires personalised individual calibration against invasive basal and post-prandial blood glucose references, which remains valid for a month. The clinical trials[65] demonstrated high accuracy with 92% of the measurements in the clinically acceptable A and B zones of the Clarke EGA. Apart from the routine diabetic monitoring device features, the device has USB and IR connectivity, and battery recharging capabilities. However, the device has yet to be commercialised as the quality of the calibration procedure and the algorithm employed for data processing need further improvement.

Sufficient penetration levels of electromagnetic waves through the body is a prerequisite for obtaining reliable readings given that the skin acts as a barrier that reflects most of these waves. Recently, MediWise (United Kingdom) reported the use of a metamaterial thin-film layer, which enables increased penetration. As electromagnetic radiation is made up of perpendicular vibrations of electric and magnetic fields, natural materials usually only affect the electric component of light (perpendicular vibrations of electric and magnetic fields), whereas metamaterials can affect its magnetic component.[62] The proposed metamaterial was shown to play a critical role in the development of a novel NI measurement of blood glucose. The device is based on high-frequency radio waves ($\sim 65\,\text{GHz}$), which can penetrate the tissue as well as providing sufficient resolution of the blood regions within. The sensor possesses an integrated nanocomposite (metamaterial) film, which temporarily renders the skin transparent to the radio waves during measurement.[63]

Temperature-regulated localised reflectance and metabolic heat conformation

The temperature-regulated localised reflectance-based NIAT involves analysis of the changes in the refractive index of tissues (mainly the skin of the forearm), which affects the scattering of light (depending upon the glucose concentration) that can then be estimated with localised reflectance signals at 590 and 935 nm.[23] However, this technique suffers from the limitation that several physiological parameters as well as disease conditions, involving fever or change in body temperature, can affect the glucose measurement.

Metabolic heat conformation-based NIAT involves the determination of blood glucose levels based on measurements of thermal generation, blood flow rate, Hb, and oxyhaemoglobin concentrations.[66] Initially, the temperature of the fingertip, ambient room, and background radiation are measured, followed by multi-wavelength spectroscopy at various wavelengths for improved glucose detection. However, the technique has only been used as an adjunct due to the high probability of interference by environmental conditions.

Optical coherence tomography

Optical coherence tomography has been used to measure glucose concentration in the IF of the upper dermis of skin in the forearm based on the delay of backscattered light compared to the light reflected by the reference arm mirror. The set-up is composed of low coherence light, an interferometer with a reference and sample arm, a moving mirror in the reference arm, and a photodetector to measure the interferometric signal resulting from the combination of backscattered light from tissues in the sample arm and reflected light in the reference arm.[23,67] As the technique exploits the scattering of light, it is quite similar to the light scatter-based localised reflectance that employs the intensity of collected light. It can obtain high-resolution two-dimensional images by in-depth (up to 1 mm depth) and lateral scanning. The rising glucose concentration increases the refractive index of the IF, thereby resulting in a change in its scattering coefficient that is used to determine its glucose concentration. Potential limitations include the sensitivity of this NIAT to varying skin temperature and motion artefacts.

Smartphone imaging and smartphone-interfaced technologies

SP-based NIATs deserve special attention as these constitute the emerging technologies for next-generation POCT, particularly given the evolution of SPs in recent years, the rapidly emerging SP applications in healthcare, and the tremendously increased number of cellphone users worldwide.[5] Current SP models are equipped with all the sophisticated device features, sensors, and capabilities that are invaluable assets for the development of prospective NIATs. SP imaging has been exploited a lot in the development of various NI devices. A wide range of smart applications for personalised healthcare have already been commercialised and are currently being used by many people. The most widely used are those from iHealth and Runtastic, the leading companies that sell personalised SP-interfaced

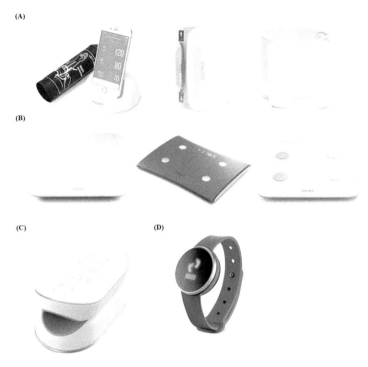

FIGURE 3.2 Personalised mobile healthcare devices from iHealth Labs Inc. for the non-invasive monitoring of basic physiological parameters. (A) (Left to right) iHealth Ease blood pressure monitor, Wireless blood pressure monitor, and Wireless blood pressure wrist monitor (B) iHealth Lite wireless scale, Wireless body analysis scale, and iHealth Core wireless body composition scale. (C) Wireless pulse oximeter (D) iHealth Edge activity and sleep tracker.

devices and smart applications for monitoring various physiological parameters such as blood pressure, heart rate, physical activity, weight, body analysis and blood oxygen saturation (Fig. 3.2 and 3.3). Most of these devices are CE marked, and FDA approved and can be purchased off the shelf at highly affordable prices within the reach of the general population. Ongoing research efforts are inclined towards the development of NIATs directly integrated into wearable technologies such as smart watches, which are considered the next generation in personalised healthcare devices.

CHALLENGES

Table 3.2 highlights key advantages and disadvantages of different NI glucose measurement techniques. The key challenges in the

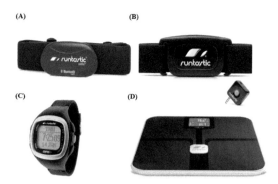

FIGURE 3.3 Personalised mobile healthcare devices from Runtastic for the non-invasive monitoring of basic physiological parameters. (A) Bluetooth low energy chest strap of the Runtastic Heart Rate Combo Monitor. (B) Chest strap and dongle of the Runtastic Heart Rate Monitor. (C) Runtastic GPS Watch. (D) Runtastic LIBRA weighing scale. (Images are copyright of Runtastic. Reproduced with permission from MDPI.[7])

development of prospective NIAT-based devices and applications lie in improvements to analytical precision, sensitivity, signal-to-noise ratio, and calibration procedures, reduced analysis time and increased cost-effectiveness. Intensive efforts are devoted towards the development of commercially viable and clinically validated technologies; flexibility for integration into wearable technologies; and compliance with healthcare, industrial and regulatory requirements.

Most of the current NIATs for NGM are limited by their analytical precision, which poses a significant hurdle to their commercialisation. Therefore, there is a dire need to tackle this limitation at a very early stage of technology development. However, as evident from the recent research efforts in the field of NGM, analytical precision can be improved significantly by developing advanced algorithms for extracting specific signals, and through the use of multiple NIATs for better signal differentiation and higher sensitivity. Precision can be further improved by integrated machine learning and employing more effective calibration procedures to take into account the varying ambient conditions and characteristics of the site of analysis such as skin. The use of multiple integrated sensors, such as those for temperature, humidity, movement, etc., will also lead to much higher sensitivity and much better calibration given significant improvements in signal-to-noise ratio. Additionally, the SNR can be enhanced using appropriate digital filters and data treatment methods, such as ridge regression, artificial neural networks, principal component analysis and partial least squares methods. Analysis time, in addition, is dependent on the specific NIAT and therefore may be difficult to be reduced, but improvements in calibration procedures and integration of multiple sensors might facilitate further reduction in the analysis times to a certain extent. Moreover, the development of new sensor and transducer concepts could lead to critically reduced analysis times, as evident from the recent development that enables NGM in just 1 second.[21]

As reimbursement of NIAT-based devices plays a major role in the adoption of the technology by the end-users and hence its viability for commercial success, there is a significant need to make the devices highly cost-effective. Therefore, the technology needs to target disease conditions and end-user applications, which possess an existing commercial market in addition to scope for prospective applications. As an example, any prospective NIAT for diabetic glucose monitoring would have tremendous commercial potential compared to niche applications having very limited business opportunities.

Further, NIAT-based devices need to be commercially viable and clinically validated at a much earlier stage in their product development to assess if they have the desired analytical performance and are hence appropriate for the projected application. The device needs to be thoroughly tested and correlated directly with established clinically accredited methods. Moreover, taking into account the rapidly increasing trend towards smart gadgets and wearable technologies, there is a great need for the NIAT to be flexible for integration into such technologies. Lastly, any new NIAT should be developed in compliance with healthcare, industrial and regulatory requirements at an appropriate stage in the technology development.

The inherent lack of specificity, in particular, NGM technologies, the weak signal, and interference from absorption and scattering by other tissue components are some of the other issues that need to be addressed. There are also several other obstacles that still need to be resolved, including the establishment of a relationship between blood glucose and glucose levels in the fluid surrounding the cells in the skin and subcutaneous tissue. Glucose levels at different body sites, such as the abdomen and the forearm, for example, need to be correlated. The ongoing research efforts by many groups will indeed provide the essential tools to tackle these challenges in NGM given significant recent advances in the field despite all these difficulties and concerns associated with the technology.

CONCLUSIONS AND FUTURE TRENDS

There have been tremendous developments in NIATs that have led to a plethora of highly prospective NGM devices for POCT. While many of these will be highly useful for healthcare monitoring and management, the most predominant application remains that of POCT non-invasive glucose monitoring for diabetic control given the rapidly increasing number of diabetics and established surplus market size. A painless NGM device will enable diabetics to monitor their blood glucose more frequently, thereby obviating or preventing harmful diabetic complications.

Numerous advances and continuous developments in NIATs have led to increased expectations and the possibility of finding prospective NI solutions to a broad range of applications. However, this substantiates the need for more intensive and highly focused research efforts to develop robust NIAT-based devices, which require substantial recurring funding that often can only be afforded by the industrial giants, such as Apple, Samsung, Abbott, LifeScan, Bayer or Roche.

The current trend is inclined very strongly towards mH and personalised monitoring devices, especially those based on smartphone and wearable technologies such as smart watches. It is anticipated that the next few years will witness many revolutionary changes in personalised healthcare monitoring and the emergence of new concepts for healthcare delivery as mH technologies make their way into the consumer market. This will generate substantial business opportunities, considering the enormous reach of such gadget-based technologies. Many general healthcare products based on smartphone monitoring, such as those for monitoring basic physiological parameters, have already been commercialised and are currently being used by millions of people. Fitness applications in smart watches, for example, are experiencing unprecedented sales growth, and catalysing increased healthcare awareness. Advances in NIAT and adapting them to the evolving trend in mH are therefore expected to lead to the development of prospective NI devices with promising applications in POCT. With continuing advances in diagnostic technology, the next generation of blood-free, painless and accurate glucose instruments will emerge in the not-so-distant future. The device will be tiny, precise and able to control an external insulin pump for daily monitoring and management of diabetes to improve the patient's quality of life. Considering the phenomenal market for NGM, the ongoing active research in this area is well positioned to overcome the aforementioned key obstacles towards the development of more precise, accurate and miniaturised glucose devices. Admittedly, the implementation of systems for NGM over 15 years ago did not revolutionise the treatment of diabetes. Considerable efforts are still needed towards the development of NGM-based continuous glucose monitoring together with an insulin pump that could culminate in an artificial pancreas system. The algorithms employed to analyse glucose measurement in the IF have also significantly improved to allow more widespread use of glucose monitoring systems.

REFERENCES

1. Zhang P, Zhang X, Brown J, Vistisen D, Sicree R, Shaw J, et al. Global healthcare expenditure on diabetes for 2010 and 2030. *Diabetes Res Clin Pract.* 2010; 87(3): 293–301.
2. Wild S, Roglic G, Green A, Sicree R, King H. Global prevalence of diabetes: estimates for the year 2000 and projections for 2030. *Diabetes Care.* 2004; 27(5): 1047–53.
3. *IDF Diabetes Atlas.* 7th ed. www.diabetesatlasorg/resources/2015-atlas html#. 2015.
4. Vashist SK. Non-invasive glucose monitoring technology in diabetes management: a review. *Anal Chim Acta.* 2012; 750: 16–27.
5. Vashist SK, Luppa PB, Yeo LY, Ozcan A, Luong JHT. Emerging technologies for next-generation point-of-care testing. *Trends Biotechnol.* 2015; 33(11): 692–705.
6. Vashist SK, Mudanyali O, Schneider EM, Zengerle R, Ozcan A. Cellphone-based devices for bioanalytical sciences. *Anal Bioanal Chem.* 2014; 406(14): 3263–77.
7. Vashist SK, Schneider EM, Luong JHT. Commercial smartphone-based devices and smart applications for personalized healthcare monitoring and management. *Diagnostics.* 2014; 4(3): 104–28.
8. Koo T-W. Measurement of blood analytes in turbid biological tissue using near-infrared Raman spectroscopy [Ph.D. thesis]: Massachusetts Institute of Technology; 2001.
9. Malin SF, Ruchti TL, Blank TB, Thennadil SN, Monfre SL. Noninvasive prediction of glucose by near-infrared diffuse reflectance spectroscopy. *Clin Chem.* 1999; 45(9): 1651–8.
10. Schrader W, Meuer P, Popp J, Kiefer W, Menzebach J-U, Schrader B. Non-invasive glucose determination in the human eye. *J Mol Struc.* 2005; 735: 299–306.
11. Kasemsumran S, Du YP, Maruo K, Ozaki Y. Improvement of partial least squares models for in vitro and in vivo glucose quantifications by using near-infrared spectroscopy and searching combination moving window partial least squares. *Chemometr Intell Lab Syst.* 2006; 82(1): 97–103.
12. Maruo K, Tsurugi M, Chin J, Ota T, Arimoto H, Yamada Y, et al. Noninvasive

blood glucose assay using a newly developed near-infrared system. *IEEE J Sel Top Quantum Electron.* 2003; 9(2): 322–30.

13. Arnold MA, Olesberg JT, Small GW. Near-infrared spectroscopy for noninvasive glucose sensing. In: Cunningham DD, Stenken JA, eds. *In vivo glucose sensing.* Hoboken, NJ: John Wiley & Sons, 2009: pp. 357–90.

14. Sibbald RG, Landolt SJ, Toth D. Skin and diabetes. *Endocrinol Metab Clin North Am.* 1996; 25(2): 463–72.

15. Monnier VM, Bautista O, Kenny D, Sell DR, Fogarty J, Dahms W, et al. Skin collagen glycation, glycoxidation, and crosslinking are lower in subjects with long-term intensive versus conventional therapy of type 1 diabetes: relevance of glycated collagen products versus HbA1c as markers of diabetic complications. DCCT Skin Collagen Ancillary Study Group. Diabetes Control and Complications Trial. *Diabetes.* 1999; 48(4): 870–80.

16. Yeh SJ, Khalil OS, Hanna CF, Kantor S. Near-infrared thermo-optical response of the localized reflectance of intact diabetic and nondiabetic human skin. *J Biomed Opt.* 2003; 8(3): 534–44.

17. Yki-Jarvinen H, Utriainen T. Insulin-induced vasodilatation: physiology or pharmacology? *Diabetologia.* 1998; 41(4): 369–79.

18. Oomen P, Kant G, Dullaart R, Reitsma W, Smit A. Acute hyperglycemia and hyperinsulinemia enhance vasodilatation in Type 1 diabetes mellitus without increasing capillary permeability and inducing endothelial dysfunction. *Microvasc Res.* 2002; 63(1): 1–9.

19. Mazarevica G, Freivalds T, Jurka A. Properties of erythrocyte light refraction in diabetic patients. *J Biomed Opt.* 2002; 7(2): 244–7.

20. Heise HM, Marbach R. Human oral mucosa studies with varying blood glucose concentration by non-invasive ATR-FT-IR-spectroscopy. *Cell Mol Biol (Noisy-le-grand).* 1998; 44(6): 899–912.

21. Kovatchev BP, Gonder-Frederick LA, Cox DJ, Clarke WL. Evaluating the accuracy of continuous glucose-monitoring sensors: continuous glucose-error grid analysis illustrated by TheraSense Freestyle Navigator data. *Diabetes Care.* 2004; 27(8): 1922–8.

22. Khalil OS. Noninvasive photonic-crystal material for sensing glucose in tears. *Clin Chem.* 2004; 50(12): 2236–7.

23. Fusman R, Rotstein R, Elishkewich K, Zeltser D, Cohen S, Kofler M, et al. Image analysis for the detection of increased erythrocyte, leukocyte and platelet adhesiveness/aggregation in the peripheral blood of patients with diabetes mellitus. *Acta Diabetol.* 2001; 38(3): 129–34.

24. Martin WB, Mirov S, Venugopalan R. Using two discrete frequencies within the middle infrared to quantitatively determine glucose in serum. *J Biomed Optics.* 2002; 7(4): 613–7.

25. Shen Y, Davies A, Linfield E, Elsey T, Taday P, Arnone D. The use of Fourier-transform infrared spectroscopy for the quantitative determination of glucose concentration in whole blood. *Phys Med Biol.* 2003; 48(13): 2023.

26. Brancaleon L, Bamberg MP, Sakamaki T, Kollias N. Attenuated total

reflection–Fourier transform infrared spectroscopy as a possible method to investigate biophysical parameters of stratum corneum in vivo. *J Invest Dermatol.* 2001; 116(3): 380–6.

27. Roychoudhury P, Harvey LM, McNeil B. At-line monitoring of ammonium, glucose, methyl oleate and biomass in a complex antibiotic fermentation process using attenuated total reflectance-mid-infrared (ATR-MIR) spectroscopy. *Anal Chim Acta.* 2006; 561(1): 218–24.

28. Laser device detects blood glucose levels without the finger-prick. www.gizmagcom/laser-blood-glucose-level-mesurement/33466/. 2014.

29. Thennadil SN, Rennert JL, Wenzel BJ, Hazen KH, Ruchti TL, Block MB. Comparison of glucose concentration in interstitial fluid, and capillary and venous blood during rapid changes in blood glucose levels. *Diabetes Technol Ther.* 2001; 3(3): 357–65.

30. Cohen O, Fine I, Monashkin E, Karasik A. Glucose correlation with light scattering patterns: a novel method for non-invasive glucose measurements. *Diabetes Technol Ther.* 2003; 5(1): 11–17.

31. Wickramasinghe Y, Yang Y, Spencer SA. Current problems and potential techniques in in vivo glucose monitoring. *J Fluoresc.* 2004; 14(5): 513–20.

32. Leboulanger B, Guy RH, Delgado-Charro MB. Reverse iontophoresis for non-invasive transdermal monitoring. *Physiol Meas.* 2004; 25(3): R35–50.

33. Kurnik RT, Oliver JJ, Waterhouse SR, Dunn T, Jayalakshmi Y, Lesho M, et al. Application of the mixtures of experts algorithm for signal processing in a noninvasive glucose monitoring system. *Sens Actuators B Chem.* 1999; 60(1): 19–26.

34. Pitzer KR, Desai S, Dunn T, Edelman S, Jayalakshmi Y, Kennedy J, et al. Detection of hypoglycemia with the GlucoWatch biographer. *Diabetes Care.* 2001; 24(5): 881–5.

35. Tierney MJ, Jayalakshmi Y, Parris NA, Reidy MP, Uhegbu C, Vijayakumar P. Design of a biosensor for continual, transdermal glucose monitoring. *Clin Chem.* 1999; 45(9): 1681–3.

36. Tierney MJ, Tamada JA, Potts RO, Jovanovic L, Garg S, Team CR. Clinical evaluation of the GlucoWatch® biographer: a continual, non-invasive glucose monitor for patients with diabetes. *Biosens Bioelectron.* 2001; 16(9): 621–9.

37. Panchagnula R, Pillai O, Nair VB, Ramarao P. Transdermal iontophoresis revisited. *Curr Opin Chem Biol.* 2000; 4(4): 468–73.

38. Park HD, Lee KJ, Yoon HR, Nam HH. Design of a portable urine glucose monitoring system for health care. *Comput Biol Med.* 2005; 35(4): 275–86.

39. Tsalikian E, Beck RW, Tamborlane WV, Chase P, Buckingham BA, Weinzimer SA, et al. Accuracy of the GlucoWatch G2 Biographer and the continuous glucose monitoring system during hypoglycemia: Experience of the Diabetes Research in Children Network. *Diabetes Care.* 2004; 27(3): 722–6.

40. Wentholt IM, Hoekstra JB, Zwart A, DeVries JH. Pendra goes Dutch: lessons for the CE mark in Europe. *Diabetologia.* 2005; 48(6): 1055–8.

41. Hillier TA, Abbott RD, Barrett EJ. Hyponatremia: evaluating the correction factor for hyperglycemia. *Am J Med.* 1999; 106(4): 399–403.

42. Ermolina I, Polevaya Y, Feldman Y. Analysis of dielectric spectra of eukaryotic cells by computer modeling. *Eur Biophys J.* 2000; 29(2): 141–5.

43. Polevaya Y, Ermolina I, Schlesinger M, Ginzburg BZ, Feldman Y. Time domain dielectric spectroscopy study of human cells. II. Normal and malignant white blood cells. *Biochim Biophys Acta.* 1999; 1419(2): 257–71.

44. Caduff A, Dewarrat F, Talary M, Stalder G, Heinemann L, Feldman Y. Noninvasive glucose monitoring in patients with diabetes: a novel system based on impedance spectroscopy. *Biosens Bioelectron.* 2006; 22(5): 598–604.

45. Pfützner A, Caduff A, Larbig M, Schrepfer T, Forst T. Impact of posture and fixation technique on impedance spectroscopy used for continuous and noninvasive glucose monitoring. *Diabetes Technol Ther.* 2004; 6(4): 435–41.

46. Caduff A, Hirt E, Feldman Y, Ali Z, Heinemann L. First human experiments with a novel non-invasive, non-optical continuous glucose monitoring system. *Biosens Bioelectron.* 2003; 19(3): 209–17.

47. Berger AJ, Itzkan I, Feld MS. Feasibility of measuring blood glucose concentration by near-infrared Raman spectroscopy. *Spectrochim Acta A Mol Biomol Spectrosc.* 1997; 53A(2): 287–92.

48. Barman I, Kong CR, Singh GP, Dasari RR, Feld MS. Accurate spectroscopic calibration for noninvasive glucose monitoring by modeling the physiological glucose dynamics. *Anal Chem.* 2010; 82(14): 6104–14.

49. Boyne MS, Silver DM, Kaplan J, Saudek CD. Timing of changes in interstitial and venous blood glucose measured with a continuous subcutaneous glucose sensor. *Diabetes.* 2003; 52(11): 2790–4.

50. Ellis DI, Goodacre R. Metabolic fingerprinting in disease diagnosis: biomedical applications of infrared and Raman spectroscopy. *Analyst.* 2006; 131(8): 875–85.

51. Baca JT, Taormina CR, Feingold E, Finegold DN, Grabowski JJ, Asher SA. Mass spectral determination of fasting tear glucose concentrations in nondiabetic volunteers. *Clin Chem.* 2007; 53(7): 1370–2.

52. Badugu R, Lakowicz JR, Geddes CD. A glucose-sensing contact lens: from bench top to patient. *Curr Opin Biotechnol.* 2005; 16(1): 100–7.

53. Cameron BD, Baba JS, Coté GL. Measurement of the glucose transport time delay between the blood and aqueous humor of the eye for the eventual development of a noninvasive glucose sensor. *Diabetes Technol Ther.* 2001; 3(2): 201–7.

54. McNichols RJ, Cote GL. Optical glucose sensing in biological fluids: an overview. *J Biomed Opt.* 2000; 5(1): 5–16.

55. Yokota M, Sato Y, Yamaguchi I, Kenmochi T, Yoshino T. A compact polarimetric glucose sensor using a high-performance fibre-optic Faraday rotator. *Meas Sci Technol.* 2004; 15(1): 143.

56. Lo Y-L, Yu T-C. A polarimetric glucose sensor using a liquid-crystal

polarization modulator driven by a sinusoidal signal. *Optics Commun.* 2006; 259(1): 40–8.

57. Lee S, Nayak V, Dodds J, Pishko M, Smith NB. Glucose measurements with sensors and ultrasound. *Ultrasound Med Biol.* 2005; 31(7): 971–7.

58. Khalil OS. Non-invasive glucose measurement technologies: an update from 1999 to the dawn of the new millennium. *Diabetes Technol Ther.* 2004; 6(5): 660–97.

59. March W, Lazzaro D, Rastogi S. Fluorescent measurement in the non-invasive contactlens glucose sensor. *Diabetes Technol Ther.* 2006; 8(3): 312–17.

60. Moschou EA, Sharma BV, Deo SK, Daunert S. Fluorescence glucose detection: advances toward the ideal in vivo biosensor. *J Fluoresc.* 2004; 14(5): 535–47.

61. Sandby Møller J, Poulsen T, Wulf HC. Influence of epidermal thickness, pigmentation and redness on skin autofluorescence. *Photochem Photobiol.* 2003; 77(6): 616–20.

62. Metamaterials. www.iop.org/resources/topic/archive/metamaterials/. 2015.

63. Glucowise™. www.gluco-wise.com/. 2015.

64. Freger D, Gal A, Raykhman AM. Device for non-invasively measuring glucose. US patent application, US 6954662 B2 (Publication date: Aug 7, 2012)

65. Harman-Boehm I, Gal A, Raykhman AM, Zahn JD, Naidis E, Mayzel Y. Noninvasive glucose monitoring: increasing accuracy by combination of multi-technology and multi-sensors. *J Diab Sci Technol.* 2009; 3: 253–260.

66. Cho OK, Kim YO, Mitsumaki H, Kuwa K. Noninvasive measurement of glucose by metabolic heat conformation method. *Clin Chem.* 2004; 50: 1894–1898.

67. Larin KV, Eledrisi MS, Motamedi M, Esenaliev RO. Noninvasive blood glucose monitoring with optical coherence tomography: a pilot study in human subjects. *Diab Care.* 2002; 25: 2263–2267.

CHAPTER 4

Continuous glucose monitoring systems

Sandeep Kumar Vashist and John HT Luong

CHAPTER SUMMARY

Considerable advances in glucose monitoring during the last four decades have resulted in highly evolved blood glucose meters, non-invasive glucose monitoring (NGM) devices and continuous glucose monitoring systems (CGMS). Glucose monitoring is a prerequisite for diabetes management, enabling glucose regulation within the desired physiological level. Minimally invasive CGMS have also led to tremendous improvements in diabetic management as shown by the significant lowering of glycated haemoglobin (HbA1c) in adults with type 1 diabetes. Next-generation CGMS with advanced features including non-invasive capability will motivate users to take all preventive steps to manage this chronic disease.

Keywords: continuous glucose monitoring systems; diabetes management; invasive; non-invasive.

CONTENTS

INTRODUCTION

There have been numerous advances in continuous glucose monitoring during the last two decades. Real-time monitoring of glucose and its regulation within the normal physiological range of 4–8 mM (72–144 mg dL^{-1}) enable a diabetic to live a healthy lifestyle without harmful diabetic complications.[1] Clinical trials, conducted by the Diabetes Control and Complications Trial[2] and UK Prospective Diabetes Study,[2] attest that intensive glycaemic control in diabetics circumvents retinopathy and nephropathy, two common diabetic complications. The use of CGMS aids in controlling the formation of highly stable advanced glycation end-products (AGEs),[3,4] whose excessive formation and deposition is closely related to the development of diabetic complications.[5–7] AGEs facilitate the pathogenesis of diabetic complications by altering the structure and function of pertinent biomolecules[8] and inducing detrimental effects on various body organs and tissues.[9,10] Therefore, they act as the mediators of the glycaemic memory. Moreover, the continuous use of CGMS in diabetics facilitates a sustained reduction of glycated haemoglobin (HbA1c) level,[11–17] which represents the long-term average of the blood glucose. HbA1c has been widely accepted as a proven biomarker for long-term glycaemic control in diabetes with a recommended level of less than 7% in most adults with diabetes.[18,19]

CGMS are highly desirable in the management of diabetes, where the blood glucose levels must be maintained within the physiological range.[20-26] CGMS provide the desired critical data about the daily glucose trend, which enables healthcare professionals and patients to manage the glucose concentration and prevent the occurrence of lethal nocturnal hypoglycaemic episodes.[27] They facilitate the determination of an appropriate insulin dose by analysing the fasting and postprandial real-time blood glucose level[28,29] and visualising the effect of therapeutics and lifestyle intervention. In this context, physical activities would be highly effective in personalised diabetic management to maintain lower diabetic glucose levels. Further, the real-time CGM curve would enable the detection of unrecognised hypo- or hyperglycaemic events[28,29] together with the trend in glucose variability regarding a mean amplitude glucose excursion (MAGE) index, a gold standard in determining glucose variability.[30] Therefore, CGMS can play a potential role in diabetic management as they can prevent glucose level fluctuation, a potent activator of oxidative stress.

Blood glucose meters (BGMs),[31] based on disposable test strips and minimally invasive lancets for taking a microliter sample from a finger tip, are widely used for point-of-care glucose monitoring. Some key industrial players are Roche Diagnostics, Medtronic, LifeScan, Bayer, and Abbott. During the last two decades, there have been numerous research efforts to develop prospective non-invasive glucose monitoring (NGM) devices.[32] Such devices facilitate the CGM by alleviating the pain and suffering of diabetics associated with the repeated finger pricking for frequent blood glucose measurements. Although the advances have not led to truly robust and precise NGM devices, some promising devices based on novel NGM concepts are currently under evaluation.

There are three configurations for implantable biosensing technology: (i) a short-term intravenous sensor, which is similar to a catheter used in hospitalised patients for up to 3 days, (ii) a short-term subcutaneous sensor that is inserted into subcutaneous tissues of non-hospitalised patients for several days, and (iii) a long-term sensor that is implanted in tissues or intravenously for an extended period, months or even 1 year. Table 4.1 highlights some current technical challenges associated with three major configurations of implantable glucose biosensors.

Most current CGMS (Table 4.2, Fig. 4.1) are based on a minimally invasive glucose sensing technology, similar to that of BGMs except

TABLE 4.1 The configuration of implantable glucose biosensors and technical issues

Configuration	Prospects and technical issues
Short-term intravenous	The most acceptable route to the implementation of an implantable sensor. Applications are limited to hospitalised patients.
Short-term subcutaneous	In the form of a needle, difficult to implement. Anaesthesia is needed to alleviate pain. Several unknown factors that might affect the transport of glucose to the implanted biosensor. The sensing signal decay is problematic and requires repeated recalibration. The relationship between the response signal and actual blood glucose values is unclear. Human trials of this approach might not be justifiable.
Long term – implanted in tissues or intravenously	There is a concern about patient safety regarding clot formation or vascular wall damage. Recalibration is only acceptable if simple and infrequent.

they detect glucose in the interstitial fluid (IF) using subcutaneous sensors. However, their use is not widespread due to high costs, discomfort, limited sensor life of a few days, and frequent calibration by BGM. The extremely high cost further limits the use of CGMS to only selected clinical settings where there is an immense need to monitor the glucose level continuously. There is a strong push for persistent research in NGM-based CGMS, serving as a catalyst for more effective diabetic healthcare and management. We provide here the advances in the field of CGMS together with the technical challenges and prospects.

CONTINUOUS GLUCOSE MONITORING SYSTEMS
Invasive
Dexcom
Dexcom SEVEN® Plus

The Dexcom SEVEN® Plus (DSP)[33] (see Fig. 4.1A) is a commercialised CGMS approved by the United States Food and Drug Administration (FDA) and Conformité Européenne (CE). This miniaturised transdermal sensor uses a round wire to measure glucose in the IF continuously for up to 7 days. The sensor is attached to the skin via an adhesive patch and provides the desired clinical precision even in

TABLE 4.2 Continuous glucose monitoring systems

Company	CGMS	CGMS type	Target site	Approval	Frequency of glucose measurements	Sensor life (Days)
Dexcom	Dexcom SEVEN® Plus	Invasive	Skin	FDA, CE	5 min	7
	Dexcom G4™ PLATINUM	Invasive	Skin	FDA, CE	5 min	7
Abbott	FreeStyle Navigator®	Invasive	Skin	FDA, CE	1 min	5
	FreeStyle Navigator II®	Invasive	Skin	FDA, CE	1 min	5
	Freestyle Libre®	Invasive	Skin	CE	1 s	14
Medtronic	Guardian® REAL-Time	Invasive	Skin	FDA, CE	10 s	3
	Paradigm® REAL-Time	Invasive	Skin	FDA, CE	5 min	3
	MiniMed® 640G system with SmartGuard®	Invasive	Skin	FDA, CE	5 min	6
	iPro®2 Professional	Invasive	Skin	FDA, CE	5 min	6
Integrity Applications Ltd	GlucoTrack™	Non-invasive	Ear lobe skin	N.M.*		N.R.**
OrSense Ltd	OrSense NBM-200G	Non-invasive	Fingertip skin	CE	1 min	N.R.**
Echo Therapeutics, Inc.	Symphony®	Non-invasive	Skin	N.M.*	1 min	N.R.**
C8 Medisensors	HG1-c	Non-invasive	Skin	CE	5 min	N.R.**
MediWise	GlucoWise®	Non-invasive	Skin	N.M.*	N.M.*	N.R.**

*Not mentioned

**Not required (as it employs non-invasive glucose sensing technology) the hypoglycaemic range. The DSP, equipped with a water-resistant and battery-operated transmitter with wireless transmitting capabilities, transfers glucose-sensing data every 5 min to a handheld receiver within 1.5 metres, which could store the collecting data up to 30 days for glucose sensing and record other activities/events. The receiver also displays a trend curve for more efficient diabetic management. The company also provides diabetic management software called Dexcom® Data Manager 3 for improved glycaemic control. The accuracy of DSP with a MARD value of 16.8% is equivalent to that of the clinically accredited YSI blood glucose analyser.[34] Another study[35] showed that DSP had MARD of 18.4% and Clarke EGA of 98.3% in A+B with 91.3% in A in the euglycaemia region. The MARD in the hypoglycaemia region was 22.5% while Clarke EGA analysis was not performed in this region. Other studies reported MARD of 21.5% in the hypoglycaemia region[34] and aggregate MARD of 16%.[36]

However, it requires a sensor warm-up time of 2 h and calibration every 12 h following two initial calibrations within the first 0.5 h. The length and gauge of the sensor probe were 13 mm and 26 mm, respectively, while the cost of DSP and four sensors were US$1158 and US$349, respectively. It is the first generation of CGMS that is no longer being sold and used.

Dexcom G4™ PLATINUM

Dexcom G4™ PLATINUM (DG4P)[37] (see Fig. 4.1B) is the second generation of a compact and light-weight CE marked CGMS launched by Dexcom in 2012, which employs a very thin transdermal glucose sensor (the thickness of human hair) for CGM every 5 min. The advanced wireless capability enables an improved transmission of readings to the receiver within 6 metres. This device has higher clinical accuracy with a MARD value of 14%, compared to 16% for the DSP. In fact, its MARD value is close to that of BGMs, 10–15%. About 97% of glucose measurements are in the A and B zones of Clarke error grid analysis. The coloured screen-based receiver is equipped with a customisable alarm for hyperglycaemia (>11.1 mM) and hypoglycaemia (<4.4 mM), and for when the receiver is out of range. Additionally, there is a default alarm in case of severe hypoglycaemia (<3.1 mM). The sensor can only be used for up to 7 days and requires calibration with BGM every 12 h. Dexcom STUDIO™ data management software is provided along with this CGMS for more effective diabetic management by facilitated analysis of the glucose pattern. A 7-day multicentre pivotal study confirms higher precision in glucose measurement by DG4P (MARD 13%), compared to DSP (MARD 16%).[36]

About 82% of DG4P values and 76% of DSP values are within 20% of the YSI values.

DG4P has the same limitations as DSP as it also requires a sensor warm-up period of 2 h and calibration every 12 h after two calibrations within the first 0.5 h. The length and gauge of the sensor probe are 13 mm and 26 mm, respectively. DG4P was sold at the price of US$1198 while the four sensors were sold at US$349.

Abbott

FreeStyle Navigator®

FreeStyle Navigator® (FN)[38] (see Fig. 4.1D) is the first generation CGMS from Abbott. It has a miniaturised sensor that is inserted into the abdomen or back of the upper arm to measure IF glucose every minute. The system is compact, lightweight and waterproof, and has an inbuilt battery-operated wireless transmitter that is attached to the body via a solid adhesive pad. It transmits glucose-sensing data to a receiver within 3 metres; and, a standalone cellphone-sized compact receiver with integrated blood glucose testing that enables

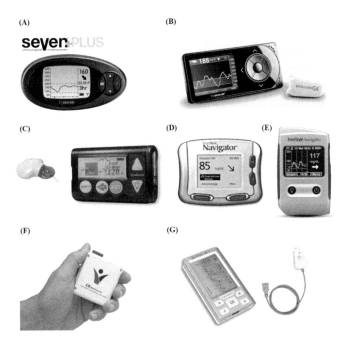

FIGURE 4.1 Continuous glucose monitoring systems. (A) Dexcom SEVEN® Plus, (B) Dexcom G4™, (C) Guardian REAL-time, (D) FreeStyle Navigator®, (E) FreeStyle Navigator® II, (F) HG1-c, and (G) GlucoTrack™. (Reproduced with permission from MDPI AG.[41])

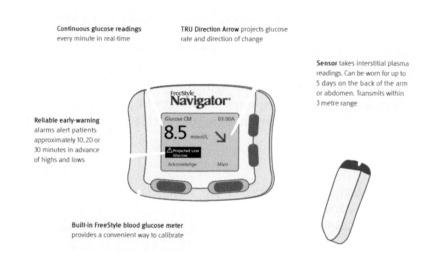

FIGURE 4.2 Visual interpretation of indicators on CGMS. (Reproduced with permission from MDPI AG.[41])

calibration via inbuilt FreeStyle BGM using test strips. Apart from providing real-time information about current glucose level every minute, the receiver's screen provides predictive information about the glucose trend. The reliable early-warning alarm in the receiver alerts the patients up to 30 min in advance if the trend points to high or low glucose levels (Fig. 4.2). FN demonstrates adequate precision as demonstrated by a MARD value comparable to that of the YSI analyser[39] with 93.7% of the readings in the clinically accurate zone of EGA.[40] Another study showed that the MARD and Clarke EGA values in the euglycaemia region were 11.8% and 98.6% in A+B with 93.7% in A, respectively,[35] while the MARD and Clarke EGA values in the hypoglycaemia region were 7.4% and 97% in A+B with 95.5% in A, respectively.[35] The warm-up time of 10 h is reduced to only 1 h in the second generation of FN.

FN has potential limitations regarding a prolonged sensor warm-up time of 10 h and the need for multiple calibrations at 10 h, 12 h, 24 h and 72 h with a built-in blood glucose meter. FN was sold at the price of US$1000 while the pack of six sensors was sold at US$375.

FreeStyle Navigator® II

FreeStyle Navigator® II (FN-II)[42] (see Fig. 4.1E) is the second generation of compact and lightweight CGMS from Abbott with better technical specifications and more advanced features. It employs the same sensor as FN that measures glucose every minute and functions for up to 5 days. Its integrated smaller transmitter transmits glucose-sensing data to the receiver within 30 metres. Similarly, the receiver is smaller but has longer lasting batteries, usable for up to 2 years. It provides glucose levels every minute along with the average, low and high blood glucose levels during the past 10 min. The receiver has the same characteristic features as FN with an illuminated colour display and more simplicity. Additionally, it has an inbuilt FreeStyle BGM to enable highly precise glucose monitoring. A typical CGM curve is shown in Fig. 4.3. FN-II provides the desired flexibility and freedom to diabetics and functions perfectly while the users are taking a shower, swimming, exercising, travelling or other routine activities. Moreover, FN-II can be used under adult supervision in children (over 6 years of age) and adolescents.

FN-II has the same disadvantages as other CGMS in that it requires more frequent calibrations at 10 h, 12 h, 24 h and 72 h with a built-in blood glucose meter. Moreover, it is more expensive than FN as it is priced at US$1524 while a sensor is available at US$64.

FreeStyle Libre®

FreeStyle Libre® is a water-resistant CGMS launched by Abbott in late 2014, which employs a small sensor patch that automatically measures glucose in just 1 s and performs CGM.[43] A small watch-shaped sensor patch (having very sticky adhesive) is placed onto the upper arm via a simple applicator, followed by scanning the sensor using a FreeStyle Libre reader® and visualising the glucose measurement reading on the reader's screen. The mobile-sized receiver with touchscreen shows the real-time glucose reading, the glucose readings of the last 8 h and a trend arrow indicating 'up or down' glucose level. However, the sensor needs to be scanned at least once every 8 h to get all CGM

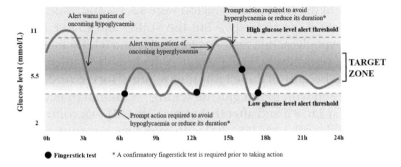

FIGURE 4.3 A characteristic continuous glucose monitoring curve and its interpretation. (Reproduced with permission from MDPI AG.[41])

data for a complete glycaemic picture. The scanning works fine even with the clothes on. The extended sensor life of 14 days is a unique feature of the device, which is approved for sales in Europe but has not yet been approved for the US market. The insertion of the sensor is very simple and does not require any preliminary training. FreeStyle Libre® is factory-calibrated and does not require constant calibration by BGM using test strips. The device is considered as the next generation of glucose meter, where the requirement of test strips and lancets has been eliminated. The device's precision in glucose measurements is equivalent to that of DG4P sensor. However, as it involves scanning of the sensor, the device does not have an alarm to alert any changes in glycaemic profile.

Medtronic

The Guardian® REAL-Time (GRT)[44-46] (see Fig. 4.1C) is a CGMS of Medtronic, consisting of a wireless transmitter attached to a transdermal sensor that measures the IF glucose levels every 10 s and transmits the results to a receiver every 5 min. A sensor can last for 6 days, and the receiver has the same characteristic features, such as prediction of trends and alerts, as described for the FN-II. The length and gauge size of the sensor were 14 mm and 23 mm, respectively. GRT is reasonably accurate with decreased hypoglycaemic excursions. The use of GRT provides an improved glycaemic control in diabetics,[14] as demonstrated by the reduction in HbA1c level after 1 month and 3 months. Another study also shows significantly improved HbA1c values just within 3 months of use of GRT in type 1 diabetics.[47] GRT is also safe to use in critically ill children and has high precision, as 99.6% measurements are in the A+B zones of Clarke EGA with the MARD value of 17.6%.[48] However, the mean absolute relative error between BGM and GRT readings is 21.3%.[49] A study showed that the MARD and Clarke EGA values in the euglycaemia region were 13.3% and 98.9% in A+B with 91.3% in A, respectively.[35] But the MARD and Clarke EGA values in the hypoglycaemia region were 13.8% and 84.4% in A+B with 81.9% in A, respectively.[35] GRT is not as deployable in intensive care unit patients because of the lengthy time required for electrode wetting and calibration with blood glucose testing.[50] Calibration needs to be performed at 2 h, 8 h and after that every 12 h. GRT was commercially available at the price of US$1400 with each sensor costing US$50.

The second generation CGMS launched by Medtronic in 2006 is the Minimed Paradigm® REAL-time Revel™ (MPRTR) system, equipped with an insulin pump to provide better glycaemic control. MPRTR, interfaced with CareLink™ personal therapy management software, provides the desired stored information about glucose levels, meals and insulin to healthcare professionals. The Bolus® Wizard calculator in the insulin pump[51] enables a tight glycaemic control by adjusting the insulin dose in response to the glucose level.

The improved CGMS MiniMed® 640G system with SmartGuard® was launched by Medtronic in 2010. It comprises a CGMS, having a new-generation Enlite™ glucose sensor and Guardian™ 2 link transmitter, and an integrated insulin pump. The glucose readings are taken every 5 min while the glucose sensor needs to be changed every 6 days. Moreover, it is interfaced with CareLink™ personal therapy management software, as used in the previous CGMS, thereby enabling the accurate tracking of glucose levels and insulin usage.

iPro®2 Professional was the new generation CGMS launched by Medtronic in 2010 mainly aimed at physicians to empower them for more effective diabetic management. It comprises a small, light and water-resistant device, a wearable CGM sensor/data logger and a docking station. It enables the patient to record and store 288 glucose readings over 24 h, which is uploaded to the web-based CareLink™ iPro software that provides easy-to-read analysis of glucose readings.

Non-invasive
Integrity Applications Ltd
GlucoTrack™[52] (see Fig. 4.1G) is the CE-approved non-invasive CGMS (NI-CGMS) developed by Integrity Applications Ltd., Israel. The compact and lightweight NI-CGMS device employs three different NGM techniques: ultrasonic, electromagnetic and heat capacity.[53] The device provides increased accuracy in the determination of blood glucose by minimising the interference effect. The procedure involves the attachment of a personal ear clip equipped with NGM sensors and calibration electronics to the ear lobe where the blood supply is abundant. The CGMS has all the desired features such as internal memory, alerts for glycaemic variations, large screen, rechargeable battery, connectivity (USB and IR), multiuser access, and software-based data processing, analysis and management. However, the device requires a personalised calibration each month against invasive basal and postprandial blood glucose. It exhibits adequate clinical precision against BGM as 92% measurements were in the A+B zones with 50% in the A zone of Clarke EGA.[54] However, it is expensive, priced at US$1926. Moreover, it requires individual calibration against basal and postprandial blood glucose references by invasive measurement. Further, the analytical performance requires significant improvement in accuracy by better calibration and improved data processing.

OrSense

The OrSense NBM-200G[55] is a CE-approved portable NGM-based CGMS, which measures glucose, haemoglobin and oxygen saturation based on the principle of red-near infrared (NIR) occlusion spectroscopy.[56] The procedure involves temporary cessation of the blood flow at the fingertip using projected light at 610 nm and 810 nm, which enhances the red-NIR signal, thereby improving the signal-to-noise ratio. The device measures glucose in a minute and is equipped with all desired features such as an easy-to-read display, alarm alerts, trends in glucose measurements, internal memory and wireless telemetry. It enables CGM for a day without requiring frequent calibration and is safe for use by patients without any contamination risk. The device's precision, obtained from over 400 subjects, is comparable to that of BGMs. A clinical trial, conducted at the Sheba Medical Center, Israel, further confirms that 95.3% of glucose measurements are in the A+B zones while 4.7% are in the C+D zones of the Clarke EGA.

Echo Therapeutics, Inc.

Symphony®[57] is an NGM-based CGMS developed by Sontra Medical Corporation, which merged with Echo Therapeutics, Inc., a specialty transdermal therapeutics company, in 2007. The glucose measurement procedure involves skin permeation via a unique transdermal permeation system known as Prelude® SkinPrep. After a brief warm-up period, a glucose biosensor is used for measuring glucose every minute on the permeated site,[32] and the data are transmitting to a remote monitor equipped with an alarm for alerting any glucose levels beyond the normal range. The device has adequate performance in the clinical trials conducted in 2011 without causing noticeable skin irritation, and the results agree well with those obtained by the YSI 2300 STAT Plus analyser and BGM. The device accuracy was reported by the company in 2012, with 96.9% of the measurements in the A+B zones of the Clarke EGA. The testing of the CGMS in diabetics, patients undergoing cardiac surgery and healthy volunteers further show adequate precision in measurement.[54] In diabetics, 89.6% and 9% glucose readings were in the Clarke EGA A and B zones, respectively. The patients undergoing cardiac surgery showed 86.4% readings in A and 13.6% readings in B zones of Clarke EGA. By comparison, the healthy volunteers showed 89.9% readings in A and 10.1% in B zones of Clarke EGA.

C8 MediSensors

HG1-c[58] (see Fig. 4.1F) is a compact and water-resistant CE-approved

NGM-based CGMS developed by C8 MediSensors (San Jose, California, USA),[32] which measures glucose with high precision in 3 min. The device employs Raman spectroscopy for glucose detection by transmitting a pulse of monochromatic light into the skin followed by detection of scattered light. The distinct Raman signature of glucose is screened out by advanced regression analysis techniques. The device contains a miniaturised glucose sensor that is worn on the abdomen via an adjustable band to provide glucose measurement every 5 min without any requirement for frequent recalibration. CGM data are transmitted continuously to an attached smartphone, which visualises the transmitted CGM data of the last 3 h instantaneously and stores the collected CGM data of up to the last 4 months. Additionally, it enables users to set up customised alerts for glycaemic variations. The cost of continuous glucose determination is lower compared to the fingerpicking test, 3 per day over 4 years. Despite raising an investment funding of US$24 million in 2012, the investment by GE Healthcare and other investors, and the scheduled product launch in Europe in 2013, C8 MediSensors ceased to function in early 2013 due to unknown reasons. The analysis of the device's precision shows 92% of glucose measurements in the A+B zones and 52% in A zone of Clarke's EGA.[59] However, the acceptable CGMS standards require at least 97% measurements to be in the A+B zones and more than 73% values in the A zone of Clarke's EGA.[44] Moreover, the upfront cost of HG1-c was placed at US$4000, well above the reach of most people.

CHALLENGES

The existing CGMS devices require significant improvements in precision, cost-effectiveness, response time and calibration.[60] The clinical accuracy of CGMS should be evaluated stringently as per the guidelines and standards of EGA[61,62] and the International Organization for Standardization (ISO).[63] Moreover, the glucose measurements provided by CGMS devices should correlate well with those performed using the established BGMs and the clinically accredited analysers with MARD values of less than 15%.[64] To date, CGMS cannot outperform or match the accuracy and analytical performance of BGMs and clinical analysers.[65-67] However, they provide extensive information about the glucose profile and trends, which enable healthcare professionals to develop strategies or interventions for more efficient diabetic management.

CGMS are very expensive with high operation costs and must be performed by a healthcare professional.[68] Therefore, the cost of CGMS is not being reimbursed by the insurance companies for most users except for selected clinical cases where their use is critically desired.[12] It remains to be seen if low-cost, but high-quality CGMS are feasible for improved commercial and healthcare viability.

The time lag between the blood glucose and glucose concentration in the IF (or tissue glucose) is another important issue. However, the time lag can be induced by the measurement time taken by the CGMS, which is dependent on the glucose trend, patient characteristics and the measurement site. Thus, a clinically validated correlation is needed to relate the blood glucose concentration with the prevalent IF glucose level. Of note is a dynamic concentration correction (DCC)-based calibration procedure[69] for determining the blood glucose level from the IF glucose level.

Most of the invasive CGMS have shown the desired analytical performance with critically reduced response time, a shortcoming of the NGM-based CGMS. There is also the need to develop prospective NGM techniques-based wearable CGMS devices, preferably in the form of smart watches or wearable bands, with the desired clinical accuracy. The recent development of GlucoWise®, an NGM device by MediWise (UK) scheduled to be launched in 2016, is a promising advance.[70] The device is based on novel NGM technology involving integrated nanocomposite (metamaterial) film and high-frequency radio waves (~ 65 GHz). But it remains to be seen if it can achieve the desired clinical accuracy in future ongoing trials and evaluation studies.

A Raman spectroscopy-based NGM device[71] for the measurement of glucose in the IF has been demonstrated by researchers at Massachusetts Institute of Technology (USA). It involves a DCC-based calibration procedure, based on the rate of glucose diffusion from the blood into the IF,[64] to predict the blood glucose concentration from the glucose levels in the IF. Similarly, a portable NGM device enabling glucose measurement in 1 s has also been demonstrated by researchers at the University of Missouri-St. Louis (USA) based on the concept of NIR spectroscopy.[72] However, clinical accuracy and correlation with established and clinically accredited technologies have not been demonstrated.

There has been extensive evidence, obtained from numerous studies such as the Juvenile Diabetes Research Foundation (JRDF) CGM trial,[73] which states that CGMS lead to much better health outcomes in diabetics.[21,23,74–85] CGMS provides the mean for keeping glucose levels within the acceptable range, preventing glycaemic variability, reducing the time spent in hypoglycaemia and hyperglycaemia, and lowering the HbA1c level. The improvements such as the reduced HbA1c level can be sustained, even for several months.[12–16,82] The real-time CGM data also enable users and healthcare professionals to decide on an effective therapeutic regimen and improved glucoregulatory exercises.[86] However, due to the lack of extensive studies, the use of CGMS is still questionable in children (under 8 years). Moreover, there is a need to develop essential skills in healthcare professionals and patients for the interpretation of CGM data.[87] Other challenges include the requirement of calibration by BGM, the need to change the transdermal glucose sensor after a few days, an elaborate operation procedure, patient discomfort and skin irritation.

CONCLUSIONS

All the research efforts to date aimed at finding a cure for diabetes have not been successful. The frequent monitoring of glucose and keeping it sustained within the acceptable physiological range is the only way for diabetics to prevent themselves from harmful diabetic complications. These actions would also be useful to those affected by impaired glucose tolerance, who carry a high risk of being diabetic in the near future. The use of CGMS will thus prevent or delay the onset of diabetes. However, the current generation of CGMS devices requires considerable improvements regarding precision, simplicity, cost-effectiveness and response time, developments which require consistent effort and continued funding that can only be afforded by big companies. Additionally, CGMS is only approved as an adjunct device, not as a replacement for BGM, and is used by a limited number of diabetics based on justified need. However, the advantages associated with extensive CGM data and trend prediction result in better health outcomes, as is well recognised by the scientific and healthcare professionals. Therefore, this substantiates the need for focused research efforts towards the development of clinically and industrially viable CGMS. The combination of CGMS with an insulin pump in closed-loop systems might also be useful for more efficient diabetic management. The development of an NGM-based NGMS device for diabetics, preferably smartphone or smart watch based, has been a vision for the last two decades. Such next-generation CGMS will motivate users to take the essential preventive healthcare interventions to control diabetes.

Considering substantial industrial investment, academic interest, and media attention, implementation of a non-invasive glucose sensor is feasible, but detection specificity still poses some technical challenges. The cost of manufacture is another deciding factor for patients in developing countries. Diabetics are always enthusiastic about the possibility of a reliable and affordable CGM device, but they have waited for a long time and wondered if such a sensor is soon available in the clinical market.

REFERENCES

1. Aronson D. Hyperglycemia and the pathobiology of diabetic complications. *Adv Cardiol*. 2008; 45: 1–16.
2. Skyler JS. The economic burden of diabetes and the benefits of improved glycemic control: the potential role of a continuous glucose monitoring system. *Diabetes Technol Ther*. 2000; 2 Suppl 1: S7–S12.
3. Forbes JM, Soldatos G, Thomas MC. Below the radar: advanced glycation end products that detour 'around the side': is HbA1c not an accurate enough predictor of long term progression and glycaemic control in diabetes? *The Clinical Biochemist Reviews/Australian Association of Clinical Biochemists*. 2005; 26(4): 123.
4. Monnier VM, Bautista O, Kenny D, Sell DR, Fogarty J, Dahms W, et al. Skin collagen glycation, glycoxidation, and crosslinking are lower in subjects with long-term intensive versus conventional therapy of type 1 diabetes: relevance of glycated collagen products versus HbA1c as markers of diabetic complications. DCCT Skin Collagen Ancillary Study Group. Diabetes Control and Complications Trial. *Diabetes*. 1999; 48(4): 870–80.
5. Schleicher ED, Wagner E, Nerlich AG. Increased accumulation of the glycoxidation product N(epsilon)-(carboxymethyl)lysine in human tissues in diabetes and aging. *J Clin Invest*. 1997; 99(3): 457–68.
6. Tsukushi S, Katsuzaki T, Aoyama I, Takayama F, Miyazaki T, Shimokata K, et al. Increased erythrocyte 3-DG and AGEs in diabetic hemodialysis patients: role of the polyol pathway. *Kidney Int*. 1999; 55(5): 1970–6.
7. Kilhovd BK, Giardino I, Torjesen PA, Birkeland KI, Berg TJ, Thornalley PJ, et al. Increased serum levels of the specific AGE-compound methylglyoxal-derived hydroimidazolone in patients with type 2 diabetes. *Metabolism*. 2003; 52(2): 163–7.
8. Vlassara H, Palace MR. Diabetes and advanced glycation endproducts. *J Intern Med*. 2002; 251(2): 87–101.
9. Meerwaldt R, Links T, Zeebregts C, Tio R, Hillebrands JL, Smit A. The clinical relevance of assessing advanced glycation endproducts accumulation in diabetes. *Cardiovasc Diabetol*. 2008; 7(1): 29.
10. McCarter RJ, Hempe JM, Gomez R, Chalew SA. Biological variation in HbA1c predicts risk of retinopathy and nephropathy in type 1 diabetes. *Diabetes Care*. 2004; 27(6): 1259–64.
11. Salardi S, Zucchini S, Santoni R, Ragni L, Gualandi S, Cicognani A, et al. The

glucose area under the profiles obtained with continuous glucose monitoring system relationships with HbAlc in pediatric type 1 diabetic patients. *Diabetes Care.* 2002; 25(10): 1840–4.

12. Blevins TC, Bode BW, Garg SK, Grunberger G, Hirsch IB, Jovanovic L, et al. Statement by the American Association of Clinical Endocrinologists Consensus Panel on continuous glucose monitoring. *Endocr Pract.* 2010; 16(5): 730–45.

13. Petrovski G, Dimitrovski C, Milenkovic T. Clinical performance of continuous glucose monitoring system in type 1 diabetics. *Diabeto Croat.* 2004; 33: 125–9.

14. Deiss D, Bolinder J, Riveline JP, Battelino T, Bosi E, Tubiana-Rufi N, et al. Improved glycemic control in poorly controlled patients with type 1 diabetes using real-time continuous glucose monitoring. *Diabetes Care.* 2006; 29(12): 2730–2.

15. Allen NA, Fain JA, Braun B, Chipkin SR. Continuous glucose monitoring counseling improves physical activity behaviors of individuals with type 2 diabetes: a randomized clinical trial. *Diabetes Res Clin Pract.* 2008; 80(3): 371–9.

16. Bode BW, Gross TM, Thornton KR, Mastrototaro JJ. Continuous glucose monitoring used to adjust diabetes therapy improves glycosylated hemoglobin: a pilot study. *Diabetes Res Clin Pract.* 1999; 46(3): 183–90.

17. The Diabetes Control and Complications Trial Research Group. The effect of intensive treatment of diabetes on the development and progression of long-term complications in insulin-dependent diabetes mellitus. *N Engl J Med.* 1993; 329(14): 977–86.

18. American Diabetes Association. Standards of medical care in diabetes – 2008. *Diabetes Care.* 2008; 31: S12.

19. Rahbar S. The discovery of glycated hemoglobin: a major event in the study of nonenzymatic chemistry in biological systems. *Ann N Y Acad Sci.* 2005; 1043(1): 9–19.

20. Vazeou A. Continuous blood glucose monitoring in diabetes treatment. *Diabetes Res Clin Pract.* 2011; 93 Suppl 1: S125–S30.

21. Girardin CM, Huot C, Gonthier M, Delvin E. Continuous glucose monitoring: a review of biochemical perspectives and clinical use in type 1 diabetes. *Clin Biochem.* 2009; 42(3): 136–42.

22. Moser EG, Morris AA, Garg SK. Emerging diabetes therapies and technologies. *Diabetes Res Clin Pract.* 2012; 97(1): 16–26.

23. Klonoff DC. A review of continuous glucose monitoring technology. *Diabetes Technol Ther.* 2005; 7(5): 770–5.

24. Sola-Gazagnes A, Vigeral C. Emergent technologies applied to diabetes: what do we need to integrate continuous glucose monitoring into daily practice? *Diabetes Metabolism.* 2011; 37: S65–S70.

25. Hovorka R. Continuous glucose monitoring and closed-loop systems. *Diabet Med.* 2006; 23(1): 1–12.

26. Hanaire H. Continuous glucose monitoring and external insulin pump: towards a subcutaneous closed loop. *Diabetes Metab.* 2006; 32(5 Pt 2): 534–8.
27. Guillod L, Comte-Perret S, Monbaron D, Gaillard RC, Ruiz J. Nocturnal hypoglycaemias in type 1 diabetic patients: what can we learn with continuous glucose monitoring? *Diabetes Metab.* 2007; 33(5): 360–5.
28. Maia FF, Araujo LR. Efficacy of continuous glucose monitoring system (CGMS) to detect postprandial hyperglycemia and unrecognized hypoglycemia in type 1 diabetic patients. *Diabetes Res Clin Pract.* 2007; 75(1): 30–4.
29. Kaufman FR, Gibson LC, Halvorson M, Carpenter S, Fisher LK, Pitukcheewanont P. A pilot study of the continuous glucose monitoring system: clinical decisions and glycemic control after its use in pediatric type 1 diabetic subjects. *Diabetes Care.* 2001; 24(12): 2030–4.
30. Monnier L, Colette C, Boegner C, Pham TC, Lapinski H, Boniface H. Continuous glucose monitoring in patients with type 2 diabetes: Why? When? Whom? *Diabetes Metab.* 2007; 33(4): 247–52.
31. Vashist SK, Zheng D, Al-Rubeaan K, Luong JHT, Sheu FS. Technology behind commercial devices for blood glucose monitoring in diabetes management: a review. *Anal Chim Acta.* 2011; 703(2): 124–36.
32. Vashist SK. Non-invasive glucose monitoring technology in diabetes management: a review. *Anal Chim Acta.* 2012; 750: 16–27.
33. Dexcom® SEVEN® Plus. www.dexcomcom/seven-plus. 2015.
34. Garg SK, Smith J, Beatson C, Lopez-Baca B, Voelmle M, Gottlieb PA. Comparison of accuracy and safety of the SEVEN and the Navigator continuous glucose monitoring systems. *Diabetes Technol Ther.* 2009; 11(2): 65–72.
35. Li G. Evaluation of continuous glucose monitoring systems. MSc Thesis, MIT, Cambridge, MA, USA. 2008.
36. Christiansen M, Bailey T, Watkins E, Liljenquist D, Price D, Nakamura K, et al. A new-generation continuous glucose monitoring system: improved accuracy and reliability compared with a previous-generation system. *Diabetes Technol Ther.* 2013; 15(10): 881–8.
37. The Dexcom® G4 PLATINUM. www.dexcomcom/dexcom-g4-platinum. 2015.
38. FreeStyle Navigator. https://abbottdiabetescarecouk/our-products/other-meters/freestyle-navigator. 2015.
39. Garg SK, Voelmle MK, Beatson CR, Miller HA, Crew LB, Freson BJ, et al. Use of continuous glucose monitoring in subjects with type 1 diabetes on multiple daily injections versus continuous subcutaneous insulin infusion therapy: a prospective 6-month study. *Diabetes Care.* 2011; 34(3): 574–9.
40. McGarraugh G, Brazg R, Weinstein R. FreeStyle Navigator continuous glucose monitoring system with TRUstart algorithm, a 1-hour warm-up time. *J Diabetes Sci Technol.* 2011; 5(1): 99–106.

41. Vashist SK. Continuous glucose monitoring systems: a review. *Diagnostics*. 2013; 3(4): 385–412.
42. FreeStyle Navigator II. https://abbottdiabetescarecouk/our-products/other-meters/freestyle-navigator-2. 2015.
43. FreeStyle Libre®. https://abbottdiabetescarecouk/our-products/freestyle-libre. 2015.
44. Keenan DB, Cartaya R, Mastrototaro JJ. Accuracy of a new real-time continuous glucose monitoring algorithm. *J Diabetes Sci Technol*. 2010; 4(1): 111–8.
45. Mastrototaro J, Shin J, Marcus A, Sulur G, STAR 1 Clinical Trial Investigators. The accuracy and efficacy of real-time continuous glucose monitoring sensor in patients with type 1 diabetes. *Diabetes Technol Ther*. 2008; 10(5): 385–90.
46. The Guardian® REAL-Time CGM System. www.medtronicdiabetescom/products/guardiancgm. 2015.
47. Tubiana-Rufi N, Riveline JP, Dardari D. Real-time continuous glucose monitoring using GuardianRT: from research to clinical practice. *Diabetes Metab*. 2007; 33(6): 415–20.
48. Piper HG, Alexander JL, Shukla A, Pigula F, Costello JM, Laussen PC, et al. Real-time continuous glucose monitoring in pediatric patients during and after cardiac surgery. *Pediatrics*. 2006; 118(3): 1176–84.
49. Bode B, Gross K, Rikalo N, Schwartz S, Wahl T, Page C, et al. Alarms based on real-time sensor glucose values alert patients to hypo- and hyperglycemia: the guardian continuous monitoring system. *Diabetes Technol Ther*. 2004; 6(2): 105–13.
50. Jacobs B, Phan K, Bertheau L, Dogbey G, Schwartz F, Shubrook J. Continuous glucose monitoring system in a rural intensive care unit: a pilot study evaluating accuracy and acceptance. *J Diabetes Sci Technol*. 2010; 4(3): 636–44.
51. Mastrototaro J, Lee S. The integrated MiniMed Paradigm REAL-Time insulin pump and glucose monitoring system: implications for improved patient outcomes. *Diabetes Technol Ther*. 2009; 11 Suppl 1: S37–S43.
52. The GlucoTrack. www.integrity-appcom/the-glucotrack/. 2015.
53. Freger D, Gal A, Raykhman AM. Method of monitoring glucose level. US Patent app. 2005; US 6954662 B2.
54. Chuang H, Trieu MQ, Hurley J, Taylor EJ, England MR, Nasraway SA, Jr. Pilot studies of transdermal continuous glucose measurement in outpatient diabetic patients and in patients during and after cardiac surgery. *J Diabetes Sci Technol*. 2008; 2(4): 595–602.
55. The OrSense NBM 200. www.orsensecom/productphp?ID=46. 2015.
56. Heise HM, Marbach R. Human oral mucosa studies with varying blood glucose concentration by non-invasive ATR-FT-IR-spectroscopy. *Cell Mol Biol (Noisy-le-grand)*. 1998; 44(6): 899–912.

57. Symphony®. http://asweetlifeorg/feature/a-non-invasive-cgm-explained-echo-therapeutics-symphony/. 2015.

58. HG1c noninvasive Continuous Glucose Monitor. www.diabeticglucosewatch. com/Diabetic_Glucose_Blog/coming-soon-hg1c-noninvasive-continuous-glucose-monitor/. 2015.

59. Lipson J, Bernhardt J, Block U, Freeman WR, Hofmeister R, Hristakeva M, et al. Requirements for calibration in noninvasive glucose monitoring by Raman spectroscopy. *J Diabetes Sci Technol*. 2009; 3(2): 233–41.

60. Rodbard D. Continuous glucose monitoring: a review of successes, challenges, and opportunities. *Diabetes Technol Ther*. 2016; 18 Suppl 2(S2): S23–S213.

61. Kovatchev BP, Gonder-Frederick LA, Cox DJ, Clarke WL. Evaluating the accuracy of continuous glucose-monitoring sensors: continuous glucose-error grid analysis illustrated by TheraSense Freestyle Navigator data. *Diabetes Care*. 2004; 27(8): 1922–8.

62. Clarke WL, Anderson S, Farhy L, Breton M, Gonder-Frederick L, Cox D, et al. Evaluating the clinical accuracy of two continuous glucose sensors using continuous glucose-error grid analysis. *Diabetes Care*. 2005; 28(10): 2412–7.

63. Klonoff DC. Continuous glucose monitoring: roadmap for 21st century diabetes therapy. *Diabetes Care*. 2005; 28(5): 1231–9.

64. Wilson GS, Zhang Y. Introduction to the glucose sensing problem. *In vivo glucose sensing*. 2009; 174: 1–27.

65. Guerci B, Floriot M, Bohme P, Durain D, Benichou M, Jellimann S, et al. Clinical performance of CGMS in type 1 diabetic patients treated by continuous subcutaneous insulin infusion using insulin analogs. *Diabetes Care*. 2003; 26(3): 582–9.

66. Yates K, Hasnat Milton A, Dear K, Ambler G. Continuous glucose monitoring-guided insulin adjustment in children and adolescents on near-physiological insulin regimens: a randomized controlled trial. *Diabetes Care*. 2006; 29(7): 1512–7.

67. Golicki DT, Golicka D, Groele L, Pankowska E. Continuous Glucose Monitoring System in children with type 1 diabetes mellitus: a systematic review and meta-analysis. *Diabetologia*. 2008; 51(2): 233–40.

68. Bartelme A, Bridger P. The role of reimbursement in the adoption of continuous glucose monitors. *J Diabetes Sci Technol*. 2009; 3(4): 992–5.

69. Barman I, Kong CR, Singh GP, Dasari RR, Feld MS. Accurate spectroscopic calibration for noninvasive glucose monitoring by modeling the physiological glucose dynamics. *Anal Chem*. 2010; 82(14): 6104–14.

70. GluciWise. www.mediwisecouk/productshtml 2015.

71. Shining a light – literally – on diabetes. http://newsmitedu/2010/glucose-monitor-0809. 2015.

72. Noninvasive glucose monitor closer to market. http://blogsumsledu/news/2011/03/29/glucose/. 2015.

73. EJDRF CDM Study Group. JDRF randomized clinical trial to assess the efficacy of real-time continuous glucose monitoring in the management of type 1 diabetes: research design and methods. *Diabetes Technol Ther.* 2008; 10(4): 310–21.

74. Klonoff DC, Buckingham B, Christiansen JS, Montori VM, Tamborlane WV, Vigersky RA, et al. Continuous glucose monitoring: an Endocrine Society Clinical Practice Guideline. *J Clin Endocrinol Metab.* 2011; 96(10): 2968–79.

75. Edelman SV, Bailey TS. Continuous glucose monitoring health outcomes. *Diabetes Technol Ther.* 2009; 11 Suppl 1: S68–S74.

76. Moreno-Fernandez J, Gomez FJ, Gazquez M, Pedroche M, Garcia-Manzanares A, Tenias JM, et al. Real-time continuous glucose monitoring or continuous subcutaneous insulin infusion, what goes first?: results of a pilot study. *Diabetes Technol Ther.* 2013; 15(7): 596–600.

77. Kestila KK, Ekblad UU, Ronnemaa T. Continuous glucose monitoring versus self-monitoring of blood glucose in the treatment of gestational diabetes mellitus. *Diabetes Res Clin Pract.* 2007; 77(2): 174–9.

78. Reach G. Continuous glucose monitoring and diabetes health outcomes: a critical appraisal. *Diabetes Technol Ther.* 2008; 10(2): 69–80.

79. Halvorson M, Carpenter S, Kaiserman K, Kaufman FR. A pilot trial in pediatrics with the sensor-augmented pump: combining real-time continuous glucose monitoring with the insulin pump. *J Pediatr.* 2007; 150(1): 103–5 e1.

80. Buse JB, Dailey G, Ahmann AA, Bergenstal RM, Green JB, Peoples T, et al. Baseline predictors of A1C reduction in adults using sensor-augmented pump therapy or multiple daily injection therapy: the STAR 3 experience. *Diabetes Technol Ther.* 2011; 13(6): 601–6.

81. Norgaard K, Scaramuzza A, Bratina N, Lalic NM, Jarosz-Chobot P, Kocsis G, et al. Routine sensor-augmented pump therapy in type 1 diabetes: the INTERPRET study. *Diabetes Technol Ther.* 2013; 15(4): 273–80.

82. Schmidt S, Norgaard K. Sensor-augmented pump therapy at 36 months. *Diabetes Technol Ther.* 2012; 14(12): 1174–7.

83. Slover RH, Welsh JB, Criego A, Weinzimer SA, Willi SM, Wood MA, et al. Effectiveness of sensor-augmented pump therapy in children and adolescents with type 1 diabetes in the STAR 3 study. *Pediatr Diabetes.* 2012; 13(1): 6–11.

84. Frontino G, Bonfanti R, Scaramuzza A, Rabbone I, Meschi F, Rigamonti A, et al. Sensor-augmented pump therapy in very young children with type 1 diabetes: an efficacy and feasibility observational study. *Diabetes Technol Ther.* 2012; 14(9): 762–4.

85. Hermanides J, Engstrom AE, Wentholt IM, Sjauw KD, Hoekstra JB, Henriques JP, et al. Sensor-augmented insulin pump therapy to treat hyperglycemia at the coronary care unit: a randomized clinical pilot trial. *Diabetes Technol Ther.* 2010; 12(7): 537–42.

86. Routen A. The utility of continuous glucose monitoring in exercise and health science. *Journal of Physical Education and Sport.* 2010; 27(2): 21–6.

87. Hammond P. Continuous glucose monitoring: the clinical picture. How to interpret and use the data. *Practical Diabetes.* 2012; 29(9): 364–8.

CHAPTER 5

Glycated haemoglobin (HbA1c) monitoring for diabetes diagnosis, management and therapy

Sandeep Kumar Vashist, Erwin Schleicher, Peter B Luppa and John HT Luong

CHAPTER SUMMARY

Glycated haemoglobin (Hb), particularly the predominant form, HbA1c, has become a primary parameter for diabetes diagnosis and a definite asset in diabetic management, for monitoring the effectiveness of the treatment regimen and the physical or other interventions taken by the diabetic. The HbA1c level over the total Hb is an indicator of the long-term average of blood glucose level in a diabetic. The lowering of HbA1c well below 6.5% and keeping it sustained for a prolonged time directly correlates with effective diabetic management, resulting in positive health outcomes to prevent or delay the onset of harmful and costly diabetic complications. However, the HbA1c test must meet stringent quality assurance, and there are no pathological conditions that preclude its clinical significance. The last decade has witnessed the emergence of several prospective point-of-care (POC) devices for the monitoring of HbA1c. The continuous improvements in POC testing (POCT), mobile healthcare (mH), smart systems and complementary technologies will lead to the next generation of smart POC devices for HbA1c monitoring, another arsenal for combatting diabetes mellitus and its sequelae.

Keywords: glycated haemoglobin; HbA1c; point-of-care devices; diabetic management; mobile healthcare; complementary technologies.

CONTENTS

INTRODUCTION

Diabetes has become an unsustainable healthcare burden and a global epidemic due to the steadily increasing number of diabetics with severe complications, which has surpassed all estimates projected by the World Health Organization (WHO) and International Diabetic Federation. This chronic metabolic disorder provokes hyperglycaemia and disturbs the metabolism of carbohydrate, protein and fat, and can be found in almost every population on the globe. The unprecedented increasing rate of diabetes substantiates the need to devise and implement more effective strategies for continuous monitoring and management of diabetes. Considering day-to-day variability in glucose and the inconvenience of measuring fasting plasma glucose, other biomarkers besides glucose have been long sought.

Glycated Hb (GHb) was discovered over 40 years ago as an 'unusual' and minor Hb component of human red blood cell (RBC) haemolysate.[1,2] Like glucose, GHb is elevated in diabetes mellitus and a predominant GHb, known as HbA1c, has been identified and advocated as the highly specific diagnostic biomarker for diabetes mellitus (DM) by the American Diabetes Association (ADA)[3] and WHO.[4] Diabetics always have higher concentrations of glycated or fast Hb as compared to non-diabetic persons[5,6] and fast Hb levels are directly related to the mean blood glucose levels and chronic diabetic complications.[7] Fast Hb is referred to as the subfraction eluted faster than the main non-glycated HbAO fraction (HbAO) in ion (cation) chromatography. This chapter focuses on the advantages and pitfalls associated with the measurement and clinical significance of HbA1c in diabetes management and therapy.

HUMAN HAEMOGLOBIN VARIANTS

Haemoglobin is a tetramer with four globin chains in red blood cells (RBC) that carry oxygen from the lungs to the body's tissues and return carbon dioxide from the tissues back to the lungs. The predominant form at birth is fetal Hb (HbF), consisting of two α and two γ chains (α2γ2) together with HbA2, a minor form of two α and two δ chains (α2δ2). The level of HbF is decreasing during childhood development and becomes a minor form in healthy adults. The most abundant form in most adults is adult Hb (HbA), consisting of two α and two β chains (α2β2). A healthy adult has approximately 97% HbA, 2.5% HbA_2 and 0.5% fetal haemoglobin. The other common Hb variants worldwide are HbS, HbE, HbC, and HbD to reflect diversified human races (Table 5.1). All of these Hb variants have single amino acid substitutions in the Hb β chain.

As discussed later, the accuracy of several HbA1c detection procedures can be affected by the presence of such Hb variants.[8] To date, the

TABLE 5.1 Some key characteristics of haemoglobin (Hb) variants found in humans

Hb variants	Characteristics
HbA	The most abundant form in most adults (over 90% of the total RBC Hb) consists of two α and two β chains (a tetramer).
HbF	Fetal Hb; the predominant species at birth, consists of two α and two γ chains. It is also present as a minor form in normal adults (< 2%)
HbA2	A minor Hb after birth with two α and two δ chains (2–5%)
HbS	Homozygosity for HbS causes sickle cell anaemia (HbSC disease)
HbE	Primarily in people from Southeast Asia. Homozygous E disease or HbEE disease is usually completely asymptomatic
HbC	HbC disease (or HbCC disease): mildly or moderately anaemic
HbD	HbD Punjab is found most commonly in the Punjab region of India

National Glycohemoglobin Standardization Program (NGSP) does not include evaluation of interferences as part of the certification programme.[9] This programme is set up to standardise GHb/HbA1c results so that clinical laboratory results are comparable to those reported by the Diabetes Control and Complications Trial (DCCT) of the UK.

MODIFICATIONS OF HAEMOGLOBIN AND DEFINITION OF HBA1C

While RBC are circulating with an average lifetime of about 120 days, the intracellular Hb is non-enzymatically modified by, for example, aldehydes or urea, leading to carbamylated Hb, and particularly by glucose that represents the major post-ribosomal modification of HbA. The modification of Hb occurs at the free amino groups; that is, at the epsilon-amino group of lysine and the N-terminus of the protein chains. The most abundant modification is the glycation at the N-terminal valine of the β-chains of Hb. This modification is 'per definition' HbA1c. The term GHb includes both HbA1c and the glycation of the free amino group on lysine residues. Although the glycation of the lysine residues is lower compared to the glycation of the N-terminal valine, HbA1c, it makes up to 3% in non-diabetic patients and is increased in diabetic patients according to their hyperglycaemia.

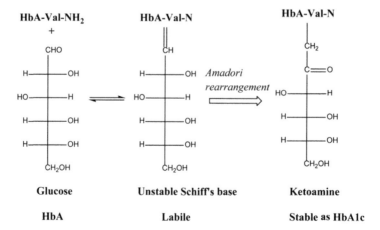

FIGURE 5.1 A two-step non-enzymatic bioanalytical procedure for the formation of HbA1c.[1] The formation is proportional to both the mean blood glucose concentration and the lifespan of the erythrocytes. (Adapted from Elsevier Ireland Ltd.)

The formation of HbA1c occurs via a two-step non-enzymatic bio-analytical procedure as shown in Fig. 5.1.[2] The first step involves the rapid formation of an unstable aldimine intermediate (Schiff's base) by the covalent binding of blood glucose to the N-terminal valine of the β-chains of Hb. Subsequently, in the second step, the intermediate undergoes a slow Amadori rearrangement into stable HbA1c with glucose conjugated to Hb.

As HbA1c is dependent on both the erythrocyte life span and the blood glucose concentration that the erythrocyte was exposed to during that time in an individual patient, the changes in the erythrocyte turnover directly affect the HbA1c value independent of the glycaemia. It is now generally accepted that RBCs live for approximately 120 days.[10] Therefore, a particular HbA1c value depicts the average blood glucose level in the subjects up to 120 days ago.[11] Nevertheless, 50%, 40% and 10% of a particular HbA1c value account for the glucose levels prevalent in the person during the previous 30, 31–90 and 91–120 days, respectively. As discussed later, this biomarker is not applicable for diabetic patients with certain haemoglobinopathies or disorders that affect the lifespan of RBC.

DIAGNOSIS OF DIABETES MELLITUS

According to the ADA guidelines,[12] the criteria for the diagnosis of diabetes mellitus have been defined (Table 5.2). These criteria are not derived from healthy cohorts (reference range) but rather from the glycaemic values from large epidemiological studies above which diabetic retinopathy may occur. Briefly, besides HbA1c, fasting or random plasma glucose values above the values shown in Table 5.2 are diagnostic for diabetes. Furthermore, a 2 h plasma glucose ≥ 200 mg dL^{-1} during an oral glucose tolerance test (OGTT) is also diagnostic for diabetes. The reference values for all glycaemic parameters are lower, and the ranges between the upper limit of the reference range and the lower limit of the diabetic range are considered as an indicator of an 'impaired glucose metabolism'. As the determination of HbA1c compared to glucose-based measurements have numerous advantages (as discussed later), HbA1c is widely used as the first parameter of choice to diagnose diabetes.

As per the ADA guidelines, HbA1c levels should be monitored at least twice per year for patients with stable glycemia and, at least, four times per year in diabetics that have high HbA1c levels or have a change in therapy. The primary objective of diabetic management based on HbA1c is to keep its concentration over total Hb less than

TABLE 5.2 Criteria for the diagnosis of diabetes (ADA, 2010).[12] (Reproduced with permission from Elsevier Inc.)

Any of the following criteria
1. *HbA1c ≥ 6.5%.*
The test should be performed in a laboratory using a method that is NGSP certified and standardised to the DCCT assay.
2. *FPG ≥ 126 mg dL^{-1} (7 mmol L^{-1} or mM).*
Fasting is defined as no caloric intake for at least 8 h*.
3. *2 h plasma glucose ≥ 200 mg dL^{-1} (11.1 mmol L^{-1} or mM) during an OGTT.*
The test should be performed as described by WHO using a load.
4. *In a patient with classic symptoms of hyperglycaemia or hyperglycaemic crisis, a random plasma glucose ≥ 200 mg dL^{-1} (11.1 mmol L^{-1} or mM)*

American Diabetes Association (ADA); Diabetes Control and Complication Trial (DCCT); National Glycohemoglobin Standardization Program (NGSP); Oral Glucose Tolerance Test (OGTT); World Health Organization (WHO).

*In the absence of unequivocal hyperglycaemia, criteria 1–3 should be confirmed by repeated testing.

53 mmol/mol or 7%[13]; that is, within the desired physiological range. The cut-off HbA1c level is not clearly established, but 5.7–6.4% is considered as the high-risk range.

Sample processing is relatively straightforward for HbA1c while it needs rigorous preparation and processing for glucose assessment, besides the fact that glucose measurement has moderate pre-analytic and biological variability versus little to no variations with HbA1c.[14] HbA1c assessment is also affected by haemoglobinopathies or diseases that increase RBC turnover. But it has been well established by several studies that tight glycaemic control is associated with fewer diabetic complications, such as cardiovascular, vision (retinopathy), kidney (nephropathy) problems[15] and neuropathy, the dysfunction of one or more peripheral nerves, typically causing numbness or weakness.

CLINICAL UTILITY OF HBA1C AND BLOOD GLUCOSE PARAMETER FOR THE DIAGNOSIS OF DIABETES

In a previous report, a population at risk for type 2 diabetes (n=2036) has been tested for both HbA1c and blood glucose parameter.[16] The OGTT classified 1523 individuals as normal glucose tolerant (NGT), 387 as impaired glucose tolerant (IGT) or having impaired fasting glycaemia (IFG), and 126 as diabetic. The 6.5% cut-off value of HbA1c classified 47% of the diabetic individuals correctly. Of the remaining 53% diabetic individuals (HbA1c < 6.5%), 35% had IFG while 65% were only diagnosed by their increased 2 h glucose values. The cut-off value of 6.5% HbA1c classified the diabetic subjects with a specificity of 98.7%. However, the sensitivity of 46.8% was low, thereby indicating that more than half of diabetic subjects are missed when using this test. Very similar results were obtained in a different cohort.[17] These results show that the use of HbA1c as the primary diagnostic test will reduce diabetes prevalence. Furthermore, it suggests that HbA1c and OGTT measurements cannot simply be exchanged, but most probably detect and define different categories of diabetes; that is, categories with different risks of cardiovascular disease.

STANDARDISATION OF HBA1C

HbA1c could not be used by healthcare professionals in clinical practice until 1993 due to the lack of a reference material for HbA1c that resulted in higher variability in measurements. However, the subsequent global standardisation of HbA1c played a crucial role in establishing the clinically accredited and analytically superior HbA1c monitoring techniques, thereby enabling the use of this novel biomarker in diabetic monitoring and management.

The most prominent role in the standardisation of HbA1c was conducted by the National Glycohemoglobin Standardization Program,[18] starting in 1996 by the American Association for Clinical Chemistry (AAAC), following the work of the International Federation of Clinical Chemistry (IFCC) working group in 1994. The standardisation of HbA1c was realised in close collaboration with and support from the commercial manufacturers, resulting in a laboratory-based reference method for HbA1c. This method consists of two steps: the enzymatic cleavage of the ß-chain yielding an N-terminal hexapeptide with or without the glycated valine. The ratio of glycated to unglycated peptide that represents HbA1c can be determined either by mass spectroscopy or capillary electrophoresis.[19] This analysis revealed that the glycation of the N-terminal valine is about 2.1 HbA1c % units lower than that previously found by chromatography-based methods. Therefore, the committee suggested using the SI units for the reference method (i.e. mmol HbA1c/mol Hb) to prevent any confusion with the value of HbA1c in mmol/L.

The standardisation of HbA1c has led to the availability of a secondary HbA1c reference material from patient whole blood, which has become the basis for the global standardisation of HbA1c methods that have been widely used by the manufacturers.[20] The HbA1c standardisation programmes were also carried out nationally by Sweden and Japan. The relations between the HbA1c levels obtained by different standardisation programmes led to several master equations[21] that enable the prediction of HbA1c values by various programs. The relationship between HbA1c and average glucose (AG) was further elucidated by the A1c-Derived Average Glucose (ADAG) study group.[22] A value of HbA1c less than the recommended cut-off point of 6.5% (48 mmol mol⁻¹) does not exclude diabetes diagnosed using glucose tests.

The HbA1c values should be reported in the same units (mmol/mol) worldwide, as suggested by ADA, IDF and the European

TABLE 5.3 The conversion table for converting the HbA1c values in mmol mol⁻¹ (currently used as suggested by IFCC) to percentages (previously used, suggested by DCCT) along with the determination of estimated average glucose (eAG) levels from HbA1c level

HbA1c (mmol mol⁻¹)	HbA1c (%)	eAG (mM)	eAG (mg dL⁻¹)
9	3.0	2.2	39
20	4.0	3.8	68
31	5.0	5.4	97
42	6.0	7.0	126
48	6.5	7.7	140
53	7.0	8.6	154
59	7.5	9.3	169
64	8.0	10.2	183
75	9.0	11.8	212
86	10.0	13.4	240
97	11.0	14.9	269
108	12.0	16.5	298
119	13.0	18.1	326
130	14.0	19.7	355
140	15.0	21.3	384
151	16.0	22.9	413
162	17.0	24.5	441
173	18.0	26.1	470
184	19.0	27.7	499

Association for the Study of Diabetes (EASD).[23] The interconversion between HbA1c (mmol mol^{-1}) and HbA1c (%) is governed by the following equation:[24]

$$HbA1c\ (\%) = 0.09148\ (mmol\ mol^{-1}) + 2.152 \tag{1}$$

The conversion table is also given in Table 5.3. Further, the estimated average glucose (eAG) can be determined from the HbA1c level by the equations (2) and (3).[22,25]

$$eAG(mg\ dL^{-1}) = (28.7 \times HbA1c\%) - 46.7 \tag{2}$$
$$eAg(mM) = (1.59 \times HbA1c\%) - 2.59 \tag{3}$$

The continuous advances during the last two decades have resulted in the development of future POC tests and devices for HbA1c monitoring and established its clinical significance in diabetes management.

HBA1C MONITORING

Routine assays

Most immunoassays rely on antibodies that recognise the structure of the N-terminal glycated amino acids (usually the first 4–10 amino acids) of the Hb β chain of HbA1c. Other HbA1c tests, based on the principles of charge difference and structural difference, have been commercialised. Ion-exchange high-performance liquid chromatography (HPLC) or electrophoresis separates Hb species based on charge differences between HbA1c and other Hb. Although capillary electrophoresis is complementary to HPLC, the electrophoresis-based HbA1c assays are no longer used in healthcare, mainly due to their

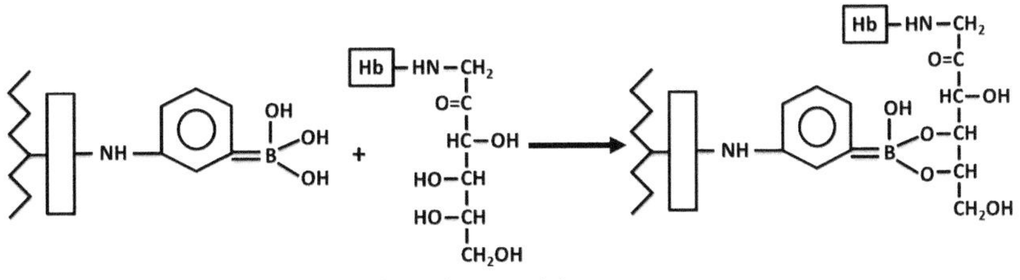

Immobilised Boronic Acid   **Glycated Haemoglobin**

FIGURE 5.2 The principle of affinity separation, which is based on the covalent binding of cis-diols of glucose in glycated hemoglobin (HbA1c) to a boronate matrix.[1] (Reproduced with permission from Elsevier Ireland Ltd.)

low throughput. Considering *m*-aminophenylboronic acid reacts specifically with the cis-diol groups of glucose of Hb, this boronate affinity method is capable of measuring total GHb (HbA1c and Hb glycated at other sites) (Fig. 5.2).

The enzymatic method is based on *Bacillus* sp. protease, an enzyme that specifically cleaves the N-terminal valine of HbA1c. Released glycated valines serve as substrates for a specific recombinant fructosyl valine oxidase (FVO) enzyme, produced in *Escherichia coli*. The recombinant FVO specifically cleaves N-terminal valines and produces H_2O_2 as a by-product. The measurement of H_2O_2 using horseradish peroxidase together with a suitable chromogen is well established in clinical chemistry. This direct enzymatic assay can be used on most automated chemistry analysers such as RocheTM Hitachi 917 series, Beckman AU (400/600/640/680), Beckman Synchron CX, LX and DXC analysers. The method is not subject to interference from the Hb variants (HbC, HbS, and HbE), carbamylated Hb, acetylated Hb, or labile HbA1c. The assay is also validated by conventional methods such as the Tosoh™ HPLC and Roche™ Tina-Quant methods. The measurement only requires a whole blood sample (ethylenediaminetetraacetic acid (EDTA) treated) of 20 mL with an assay range of 4% to 12% for HbA1c. This approach can be extended for analysis of glycated serum protein (GSP), in particular, glycated albumin, another useful indicator of diabetic management. In this case, proteinase K is used to digest GSP into low molecular weight glycated protein fragments (GPF). The second enzyme, specific fructosaminase, then catalyses the oxidative degradation of GPF to protein fragments or amino acids, glucosone, and H_2O_2.

Various clinically accredited instrument-based assays for the centralised lab have also been developed using instruments such as Bio-Rad Variant™ II Haemoglobin Testing System (based on HPLC method) and Roche COBAS INTEGRA® 800 closed tube system (based on turbidimetric inhibition immunoassay).[26] In brief, the immunologic method uses a specific antibody against the first six amino acid residues of the glycated NH_2-terminal of Hb. HbA1c causes inhibition of agglutination and decreases the measured absorbance. The COBAS INTEGRA® (Roche) uses monoclonal antibodies attached to latex particles. The change in turbidity is inversely correlated with the concentration of bound glycopeptides. More detailed information on commercial systems for the detection of HbA1c is summarised in Table 5.4.[27]

Various factors can affect the determination of HbA1c (Table 5.5). Interferences of new drugs and metabolites on Hb are unknown and

TABLE 5.4 Principles of the detection methods for HbA1c; their advantages and disadvantages

Detection methods	Advantages	Disadvantages
Ion (cation) chromatography At pH 6.9, the normal Hb has an isoelectric point of 6.87. HbA1c with a lower isoelectric point migrates faster than other Hb components.	• Commercial modern systems are highly efficient (automated, high throughput, and robust). • Meet the clinical requirements of reliability. • No significant interference from the Schiff base or carbamylated Hb (modified by urea). • In Europe, 65% of the central labs use ion chromatography compared to 30% in the USA.	• The separation of HbA1c is overwhelmed by HbAO (20-fold higher concentration). • Samples (maximum 100 specimens) can only be analysed one by one. • A stand-alone instrument in the central lab.
Affinity chromatography m-amino phenylboronic acid cross-linked on agarose (other matrices) binds the cis–diol groups of the glucose.	• The binding is specific for glycated Hb, not non-glycated Hb. • HbAO is no longer a major interfering species. • Less sensitive to temperature and interferences from carbamylated and fetal Hb.	• HbA1c must be measured together with other glycol Hb. Ionic and hydrophobic forces also contribute to this interaction. • The requirement of higher robustness for the affinity matrices, particularly the agarose gel system. • Measures not only glycation of N-terminal valine on β chain but also β chains glycated at other sites and glycated α chains. • Only 10% of the central lab in the USA uses affinity chromatography. Only a few central labs in Europe uses this technology.
Immunochemical assays A specific antibody for HbA1c is targeted against the β N-terminal glycated tetrapeptide or hexapeptide group.	• Assay design is variable: immunoturbidimetry, latex-competitive immunoturbidimetry, and enzymatic detection. • Ease of adaptation in the central medical laboratory. • 60% of the central labs in the USA vs. 35% in Europe use an immunochemical test. • Not affected by HbE, HbD or carbamylated Hb.	• A nonlinear calibration curve, i.e. the requirement of a multilevel calibration. • The reagent stability is limited (variable from test to test), relatively frequent recalibration is needed. • The total Hb must be measured separately by a different principal procedure. • Some interference with HbF.

TABLE 5.5 Factors that can affect the determination or interpretation of HbA1c.[29] (Reproduced with permission from Elsevier Inc.)

Factor	Increased HbA1c	Decreased HbA1c	Variable change in HbA1c
Erythropoiesis	• Iron deficiency • B12 deficiency • Decreased erythropoiesis	• Use of erythropoietin, iron or B12 • Reticulocytosis • Chronic liver disease	
Altered Hb			• Fetal Hb • Haemoglobinopathies • Methemoglobin • Genetic determinants
Glycation	• Alcoholism • Chronic renal failure • Decreased erythrocyte pH	• Ingestion of aspirin, vitamin C or vitamin E • Haemoglobino-pathies • Increased erythrocyte pH	
Erythrocyte destruction	• Increased erythrocyte lifespan: • Splenectomy	• Decreased erythrocyte lifespan: • Chronic renal failure • Haemoglobino-pathies • Splenomegaly • Rheumatoid arthritis • Antiretrovirals • Ribavirin • Dapsone	
Assays	• Hyperbilirubinemia • Carbamylated Hb • Alcoholism	• Hypertriglyceri-demia	• Haemoglobinopathies
Metabolic control	• Large doses of aspirin • Chronic opiate use	• Adverse metabolic control decreases erythrocyte lifespan[30]	

far from a certainty. As an example, aspirin modifies several sites, likely lysine residues, on both the α and β chains of HbA *in vitro*. Acetylated lysine residues confer a negative charge and other properties of the modified Hb. Although *in vivo* acetylation has not been confirmed, this point needs to be taken into consideration, in particular, the detection method is ion chromatography. Erythropoietin and its related substances also affect the half-life of RBC,[28] and patients with renal failure have reduced RBC survival due to anemia, which affects the quantity of HbA1c. In contrast, higher HbA1c values often occur in people with vitamin B12 or folate deficiency or after splenectomy. Similarly, iron deficiency anaemia may extend the lifespan of RBC with increasing HbA1c.

Point-of-care assays

Commercial point-of-care analysers

Several devices have been developed during the last decade for the POC monitoring of HbA1c[31] with the most prominent devices being described below and summarised in Table 5.6.

1. Clover A1C (Infopia, Kyunggi, Korea)

This quantifies HbA1c with the detection range of 4–14% in 5 min using boronate-affinity binding precipitation-based one-step assay, which uses 4 µL of whole blood (or venous blood) sample by means of a built-in capillary tip that is inserted into the analyser. The analyser has an internal memory that stores up to 200 test results and has a barcode scanner. It displays HbA1c measurements in both IFCC as well as DCCT units. The assay procedure involves the insertion of new test cartridge into the analyser, taking a 4 µL sample into the built-in capillary tip on the reagent pack, putting the reagent pack into the test cartridge, and reflectance-based optical readout. The test cartridge comprises a cartridge and a reagent pack containing the reaction and washing solutions. The reaction solution contains the chemicals, which cause the lysis of the RBC and bind specifically to Hb, and boronate resin that binds HbA1c via their cis-diols. The rotation of the blood sample mixture to the cartridge's measurement zone after the insertion of the test cartridge into the analyser enables the determination of total Hb in the blood sample by measuring the reflectance of the photo sensor light-emitting diode (LED) and photodiode. Subsequently, the rotation of the cartridge allows the washing solution to wash out the non-glycated Hb, thereby enabling the specific determination of HbA1c. The ratio of HbA1c and total Hb can then be calculated.

2. DCA Vantage™ (Siemens Medical Solutions Diagnostics, Tarrytown, NY, USA)

This enables the POC determination of HbA1c in the detection range of 2.5–14% using 1 μL of the whole blood sample. It employs an NGSP-certified latex agglutination inhibition immunoassay that takes just 6 min. The analyser has been the most widely used analyser for HbA1c analysis due to its high analytical precision and sensitivity. It has a built-in memory to store up to 4000 test measurements and up to 1000 operator names. It is equipped with a POCT1-A2 communication protocol, which enables easy and simple connectivity and automatic uploading of results to the data management systems, laboratory information systems and hospital information systems.

3. Alere Afinion™ Test System (Alere Technologies AS, Oslo, Norway)

This determines HbA1c in 3 min using an affinity separation-based assay and a POC analyser (Fig. 5.3). The NGSP-certified assay takes only 1.5 μL of the whole blood sample and detects HbA1c in the range of 4–15%. The Test Cartridge contains all required reagents and has an integrated sampling device. When the Test Cartridge enters the Analyzer, the integrated camera reads the barcode and assay processing is initiated. After processing, the reaction area is illuminated by LEDs and the reflected light is detected by the integrated camera. However, the assay only uses whole blood sample and does not work with haemolysed sample. The POC assay involves a simple analytical

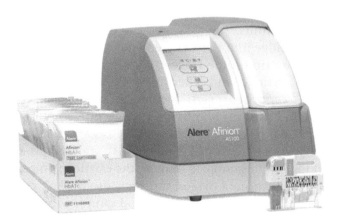

FIGURE 5.3 Alere Afinion™ point-of-care test system for HbA1c measurement, consisting of the Alere Afinion™ AS100 Analyzer and the Alere Afinion™ HbA1c test cartridges. (Reproduced with permission from Alere Technologies AS, Norway.)

procedure that involves sample uptake using a capillary sampling device; inserting the sampling device in the test cartridge, and placing the test cartridge in the analyser for assay readout.

4. NycoCard Test System (Alere Technologies AS, Oslo, Norway)

This quantifies HbA1c in just 3 min using an affinity separation-based assay procedure, which comprises four simple process steps: Hb precipitation, sample dispensing, washing, and optical readout. However, it uses only 5 μL of capillary blood or anticoagulated venous blood (EDTA, citrate or heparin) sample using a capillary tube, and does not work with the haemolysed sample. The POC assay detects 4–15% HbA1c in diluted whole blood without any interferences from various Hb variants (i.e. HbC, HbE, HbF, HbJ, and HbS) and carba-mylated Hb. The assay is performed using a portable battery-charged NycoCard™ Reader II, which comprises an optical instrument box and a reader pen (540 g).

5. In2it™ (Bio-Rad, Hercules, CA, USA)

This determines HbA1c in the detection range of 4–14% using a boronate affinity chromatographic separation-based assay that takes 10 min. It requires only 10 μL of capillary whole blood or EDTA blood sample. The analyser weighs only 0.84 kg and has dimensions of 130 mm wide × 120 mm deep × 100 mm high. The In2it™ system comprises the In2it™ analyser, the In2it™ test cartridges and an In2it™ system check cartridge. The company supplies unique blood collection devices known as blood keys. The measurement procedure involves the drawing of 10 μL of blood from the fingertip using the blood key, which is followed by putting the blood key into the test cartridge that is then placed in the analyser. The test cartridge contains several chambers for sampling, lysis, washing, elution and detection. Initially, the whole blood sample is mixed with sample buffer that contains a surfactant to lyse the RBCs, and boronate functionalised beads to bind to HbA1c. After that, the non-glycated Hb is washed away and taken to another chamber by gravity, where it is measured by taking the absorbance at 440 nm. The HbA1c bound to boronate beads is released by treatment with elution buffer containing sorbitol and HbA1c is measured by taking the absorbance at 440 nm.

The HbA1c level is calculated as follows:

$$\text{HbA1c (\%)} = M \left(\frac{[A_{\text{glycated fraction}} \times 100]}{[A_{\text{glycated fraction}} + A_{\text{non-glycated fraction}}]} \right) + C \tag{4}$$

where M is the slope and C is the intercept employed to correct the crude value.

6. Quo-Test™ (Quotient Diagnostics, Surrey, UK)

This quantifies HbA1c in just 3 min using boronate affinity separation and a fluorescent quenching-based assay. The assay requires 4 μL of whole or venous blood sample. The whole blood sample can be taken by lancing the fingertip using standard commercial lancets. The analyser is compact (205 mm high × 205 mm wide × 135 mm deep), lightweight (1.3 kg) and easy to operate. It has an internal memory to store up to 7000 results and is NGSP certified. The HbA1c measurement just involves three process steps: sample collection, insertion of sample cartridge into the analyser, and the assay readout. The POC analyser reports HbA1c levels in IFCC as well as DCCT values and detects HbA1c in the range of 4–17% (i.e. 20–162 mmol mol^{-1}). The reported imprecision of the assay is CV of less than 3% at 7% HbA1c level. Further, it is unaffected by the various Hb variants.

7. Quo-Lab™ (Quotient Diagnostics, Surrey, UK)

This quantifies HbA1c in 3 min using boronate affinity separation and a fluorescent quenching-based assay. The procedure is similar to that of Quo-Test™ but employs some manual handling.

8. B-analyst® (Menarini Diagnostics)

This quantifies HbA1c in 4 μL of a whole blood sample using a latex agglutination-based turbidimetric immunoassay that has a detection range of 3.3–12.6% and takes 8 min. However, it uses only whole blood sample and does not work with the haemolysed sample. The analyser is 340 mm wide × 290 mm deep × 270 mm high and weighs about 9.5 kg. The assay employs an advanced micro total analysis system-based chip filled with liquid reagents, which works in three stages. The first stage involves the haemolysis of RBCs and adsorption of total Hb (including HbA1c) on the surface of the latex bead. The second stage involves the reaction of adsorbed Hb with anti-human HbA1c mouse monoclonal antibody. The third stage involves the measurement of turbidity due to the formation of aggregate (immune complex) at 635 nm, and the determination of HbA1c concentration from the standard curve.

9. COBAS B101 (Roche Diagnostics)

This employs a latex agglutination inhibition immunoassay that requires 6 min for the quantification of HbA1c in the range of 4–14%

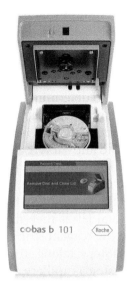

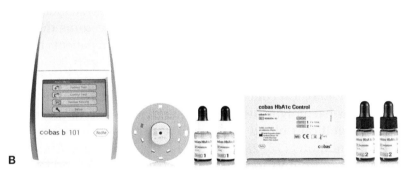

FIGURE 5.4 Schematic of the COBAS B101 point-of-care analyser-based assay for HbA1c. (A) An integrated view of analyser with HbA1c disc inside. (B) Complete view of analyser together with all assay components. (Reproduced with permission from Roche Diagnostics Ltd, Switzerland.)

using only 2 μL of the blood sample (Fig. 5.4). The assay is based on the measurement of photometric transmission, where total Hb and HbA1c are measured in separate chambers of a single test cartridge (disc shaped) at 525 and 625 nm, respectively. Once the whole blood sample from the finger prick is transferred to the HbA1c disc, it must be inserted into the analyser within 60 s. The built-in memory can store up to 5000 results, 500 quality control results and 50 operator IDs. It supports POCT1A interface protocol that enables connectivity to data management systems, laboratory information systems and hospital information systems. It can also be integrated with a barcode scanner.

10. A1CNow+ (Bayer HealthCare, Sunnyvale, CA, USA)

This uses an immunoassay to determine HbA1c in the linear range of 4–13% in 5 min. A dry reagent chemistry-based strip is used, where the addition of diluted blood sample enables the migration of blue microparticles conjugated to anti-HbA1c antibodies along the reagent strips. The HbA1c level is determined from the amount of blue microparticles that are captured on the test strip. The total Hb is determined from another portion of the test, where the sample diluent converts the Hb to met-Hb. The total Hb is then determined from the intensity of met-Hb colour on the reagent strips. The analytical procedure involves several sequential steps: taking 10 µL of the whole blood sample from the finger prick using a capillary; dispensing the sample into a sample tube pre-filled with diluent; mixing the sample by inversion; inserting the cartridge into the monitor; adding the diluted sample via a dropper to the sample port; reading the HbA1c measurement from the display screen in 5 min; and, removing and discarding the used cartridge. However, the assay gives incorrect results in patients having very high levels of HbF, HbS, HbC or other Hb variants. Moreover, decreased HbA1c levels are indicated in the case of patients affected by pathophysiological conditions associated with reduced RBC survival such as haemolytic diseases (haemolytic anaemia), pregnancy or recent significant blood loss. The test also works under limited ambient conditions (18–28°C and 15–80% humidity). There was no interference from various substances (such as triglyceride, acetaminophen, ascorbic acid, ibuprofen, acetylsalicylic acid, glyburide, metformin, and bilirubin) that were tested at five times their normal physiological levels or therapeutic doses.

11. InnovaStar® (DiaSys, Holzheim, Germany)

This employs an NGSP/IFCC certified agglutination immunoassay that takes 6.5 min for the determination of HbA1c in the range of 3–14% and incorporates individual haematocrit correction. The HbA1c test involves the uptake of 10 µL of whole blood using a glass capillary, which is followed sequentially by breaking the capillary into the sample tube, sample mixing by inversion, placing the sample tube into the loading slider, inserting the slider into the analyser, and the optical measurement to determine the HbA1c level. The analyser is equipped with a barcode scanner, weighs 4 kg and is 200 mm wide

TABLE 5.6 Point-of-care analyser-based HbA1c assays

Point-of-care analysers (manufacturer)	Assay type	Assay duration (in min)	Sample required (in µL)	HbA1c detection range
Clover A1c (Infopia, Kyunggi, Korea)	Boronate-affinity chromatography separation	5	4	4–14% (20–130 mmol mol^{-1})
DCA Vantage™ (Siemens Medical Solutions Diagnostics, Tarrytown, NY, USA)	Latex agglutination inhibition immunoassay	6	1	2.5–14% (4–130 mmol mol^{-1})
Alere Afinion™ Test System (Alere Technologies AS, Oslo, Norway)	Boronate-affinity chromatography separation	3	1.5	4–15% (20–140 mmol mol^{-1})
NycoCard™ Test System (Alere Technologies AS, Oslo, Norway)	Boronate-affinity chromatography separation	3	5	4–15% (20–140 mmol mol^{-1})
In2it™ (Bio-Rad, Hercules, CA, USA)	Boronate-affinity chromatography separation	10	10	4–14% (20–130 mmol mol^{-1})
Quo-Test™ (Quotient Diagnostics, Surrey, UK)	Boronate-affinity chromatography separation and Fluorescent quenching-based assay	3	4	4–17% (20–162 mmol mol^{-1})
Quo-Lab™ (Quotient Diagnostics, Surrey, UK)	Boronate-affinity chromatography separation and Fluorescent quenching-based assay	3	4	4–17% (20–162 mmol mol^{-1})
B-analyst® (Menarini Diagnostics)	Latex agglutination based turbidimetric immunoassay	8	4	3.3–12.6% (12.5–114 mmol mol^{-1})
COBAS B101 (Roche Diagnostics)	Latex agglutination inhibition immunoassay	6	2	4–14% (20–130 mmol mol^{-1})

(*continued*)

Point-of-care analysers (manufacturer)	Assay type	Assay duration (in min)	Sample required (in μL)	HbA1c detection range
A1CNow+ (Bayer HealthCare, Sunnyvale, CA, USA)	Immunoassay	5	10	4–13% (20–119 mmol mol^{-1})
InnovaStar® (DiaSys, Holzheim, Germany)	Agglutination immunoassay	6.5	10	3–14% (9–130 mmol mol^{-1})

× 150 mm high × 170 mm deep. It displays HbA1c levels in IFCC and DCCT units. It demonstrated good repeatability of 1.9% and 1.6% for the capillary and venous blood samples, respectively. However, the analyser has not shown the desired accuracy of more than 95% of the measurements to be within less than 10% of the results provided by the clinically accredited method.

Analytical performance

Many previous reports have clearly shown the inadequate performance of many POC analysers.[32–34] A study revealed that the six of eight POC analysers did not meet the established standard criteria for adequate analytics.[35] Only the DCA Vantage and the Alere Afinion™ had acceptable performance with a total coefficient of variation of less than 3% in the clinically relevant HbA1c range. A subsequent investigation by the same group also showed that the further improved Quo-Test analyser also partially passed the acceptance criteria.[36] Similarly, a more recent study of the same group has illustrated that DCA Vantage™, Alere Afinion™, COBAS B101 and B-analyst instruments have passed the acceptable performance criteria, while Quo-Lab, Quo-Test, and InnovaStar have achieved the precision standards but lacked the criteria for bias.[37]

DCA Vantage™ and Alere Afinion™ analyser-based HbA1c analysis was found to have high analytical performance equivalent to that of clinically accredited HPLC methods.[38,39] But it has also been reported that there are potential interferences of developed HbA1c assays with Hb variants. The inadequate performance is mainly due to the classification of existing HbA1c assays as CLIA-waived tests, which obviates the need for stringent quality control and robust analytical performance as required for the clinically accredited laboratory-based methods. A previous validation study has shown that most POC instruments have inadequate analytical performance[35] and high variability in results, which can severely impact the clinical diagnosis and decisions.

There is a need for critically improved HbA1c monitoring devices with novel assays or technologies, which can only be developed in an interdisciplinary set-up comprising clinical chemists (responsible for taking results), healthcare professionals (responsible for interpreting results), biomedical engineers and other scientific researchers. The clinical chemist would develop/screen an HbA1c method with the desired performance for clinical diagnostics and provide the health-care professionals with the desired information to correctly interpret the results and take an appropriate clinical decision. Therefore, positive health outcomes and effective diabetic management are highly dependent on the precision, accuracy, robustness and reproducibility of the HbA1c analysis method. Moreover, the responsibility of POC devices for HbA1c analysis should be assigned to and guided by the central laboratory. Other Hb variants might interfere with HbA1c measurement as pointed out by Little and Roberts.[40] Particular attention is paid to the assessment of glycaemic control in patients homozygous for HbS or HbC, with HbSC disease, or with other conditions affecting erythrocyte survival. Both the user and clinician must be aware of this limitation and select a method with minimal interference. In this particular case, the chromatogram of an ion-exchange HPLC method must be carefully inspected to identify the presence of different peaks produced by such variants. The central laboratory must be able to assess whether the Diazyme's IFCC-certified Direct Enzymatic HbA1c Assay has interference from such Hb variants as reported by the manufacturer.[41]

The measurement of fructosamine deserves a brief mention here as its level in the blood reflects glucose levels over the previous 2–3 weeks. Strictly, fructosamine is 1-amino-1-deoxy fructose or isoglucosamine, as synthesised by Fischer in 1886.[42] The term fructosamine is often referred to as glycated albumin or protein in the literature. In clinical chemistry, fructosamine is referred to as glycated protein.[43] The fructosamine level of normal subjects ranges from 205 to 285 μM. Fructosamine may be considered in the following special cases where HbA1c testing cannot be reliably measured:

- *Rapid changes in diabetes treatment* – Efficacy of medication adjustment and diet can be evaluated after a few weeks rather than months.
- *Diabetic pregnancy* – The needs of a diabetic mother frequently change during gestation.

- *Shortened RBC lifespan* – Haemolytic anaemia or blood loss.
- *Abnormal forms of Hb* – The presence of some Hb variants, e.g. HbS in sickle cell anaemia.

FRUCTOSAMINE AS ALTERNATIVE FOR HBA1C

Some key analytical procedures have been developed as shown in Fig. 5.5. The reference method for fructosamine is high-pressure liquid chromatography (HPLC), based on the hydrolysis of fructosamine by 6 M HCl at 95 °C for 18 h to lysine (50%), furosine (30%) and pyridoxine (10%). Furosine is quantified by HPLC using a reverse phase column with ultraviolet (UV) detection at 254 nm and 280 nm.[44] An enzyme assay is feasible for fructosamine but requires three different enzymes. The first step involves proteinase K to break down glycated protein to glycated protein fragments, which is subject to ketoamine oxidase to produce amino acids and H_2O_2. A chromogen is then used to determine H_2O_2 and the reaction is catalysed by horseradish peroxidase.

Colorimetric assays have been advocated for the determination of fructosamine. The serum is added to carbonate buffer (pH 10.8, 37 °C) containing nitrobluetetrazolium (NBT). Fructosamine reduces NBT under alkaline conditions, and the change in absorbance is measured at 530 nm. The NBT method is subject to a variety of interferences, and EDTA and heparin plasma samples often provide lower fructosamine results than serum samples.[45,46] Other interfering species are urate, glutathione, vitamin C, cysteine, methyldopa, dobesilate calcium, oxytetracycline and bilirubin.

Phenylhydrazine can react with fructosamine to form a phenylhydrazone adduct with absorption at 350 nm. The assay based on 2-thiobarbituric acid (TBA) is more time-consuming as the serum is heated with oxalic or acetic acid at 100 °C for 18–24 h to form 5-hydroxymethylfurfuraldehyde (HMF). After precipitation and removal of protein, HMF in the supernatant is heated with TBA at 40 °C for 30 min to form a derivative with an absorbance at 443 nm. It should be noted that fructosamine is not applicable in case there are significant abnormalities of plasma protein concentrations such as diabetes with nephrotic syndrome, liver cirrhosis, paraproteinaemias and untreated thyroid disease.

HbA1c can be fragmented to small glycated peptide fructosyl valine (FV) that is then oxidised by fructosyl amino acid oxidase. Similar to the principle of glucose biosensor technology, the reaction can be followed by oxygen consumption or hydrogen peroxide

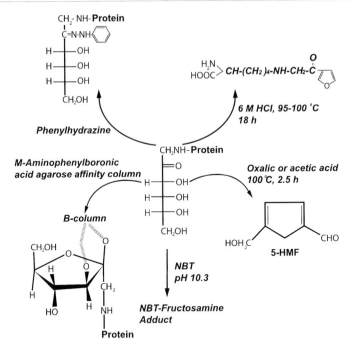

FIGURE 5.5 Various analytical procedures for the analysis of fructosamine. (Adapted from Armbruster, 1987.[42])

(H_2O_2), a by-product of the enzyme reaction. To date, several attempts have been reported for the development of a biosensor for fructosyl valine.[47] Obviously, the technology acquired for glucose sensing using glucose oxidase can be translated to fructosyl amino acid oxidase. Proteolysis of HbA1c is the limiting step and might lead to the formation of fructosyl lysine that might interfere with the detection of FV. Long response time and low storage stability are two major drawbacks of this technology. As discussed previously, the cis-diol bonds of glucose interact with boronic acids to form boronate esters, which could be determined by electrochemical impedance spectroscopy. This approach circumvents the time-consuming preliminary step to release FV from HbA1c by a protease. However, there is still a need for separate determination of the total haemoglobin content, making it an inconvenient approach. In brief, biosensing based on FV detection requires several steps for sample preparation, which prevents its widespread application in point-of-care devices.

CONCLUSIONS

HbA1c is a very useful biomarker for diabetic management as it provides an indication of glycaemic control, which is required for evaluating the effectiveness of treatment and lifestyle/nutritional intervention provided to diabetics. It has been adopted globally as an essential standard for diabetic care. The ADA has recommended to achieve and sustain the HbA1c level of below 53 mmol/mol in diabetic patients. However, most of the commercial POC assays for HbA1c have not shown high analytical performance similar to that of clinically accredited central lab assays. Moreover, it has been shown that most POC analysers have shown conflicting results. Therefore, there is a compelling need for tight quality control and high-performance criteria for POC assays, which will lead to significantly improved POC devices and HbA1c assays. The trend towards personalised mobile healthcare devices is in line with the ongoing research efforts in the field of HbA1c monitoring.

HbA1c remains as a longitudinal and significant biomarker and patients must monitor this parameter over their lifetime. As a high-volume request in the medical laboratory, the detection procedure must be fast to process high throughput of samples with high specificity and reproducibility. HbA1c is combined with glucose measurement and its relationship with glucose might be different for patients with different ages, ethnicity and geography. The analysis of glycated albumin (GA) deserves a brief mention here as this biomarker might be combined with HbA1c to provide an overall picture of the average blood sugar level over a period of weeks or months in diabetic management and control. The GA reference range is 11.9–15.8% of the USA population, in agreement with other populations[48,49] as the binding glucose to GA is 1–3. GA is not standardised, and different medical conditions also affect albumin turnover.[50-52] Like HbA1c, the applicability of GA is case specific, and this biomarker is not optimal for glycaemic control in all patients with diabetes. Affordability is another concern, in particular for diabetics of most low and middle-income countries, whereas glucose monitoring is more affordable in most countries.

REFERENCES

1. Lenters-Westra E, Schindhelm RK, Bilo HJ, Slingerland RJ. Haemoglobin A1c: Historical overview and current concepts. *Diabetes Res Clin Pract.* 2013; 99(2): 75–84.

2. Higgins T. HbA(1c): an analyte of increasing importance. *Clin Biochem.* 2012; 45(13–14): 1038–45.
3. International Expert Committee. International Expert Committee report on the role of the A1C assay in the diagnosis of diabetes. *Diabetes Care.* 2009; 32(7): 1327–34.
4. World Health Organization. Use of glycated haemoglobin (HbA1c) in diagnosis of diabetes mellitus: abbreviated report of a WHO consultation. www.whoint/diabetes/publications/report-hba1c_2011pdf. 2011.
5. Rahbar S. An abnormal hemoglobin in red cells of diabetics. *Clin Chim Acta.* 1968; 22(2): 296–8.
6. Rahbar S, Blumenfeld O, Ranney HM. Studies of an unusual hemoglobin in patients with diabetes mellitus. *Biochem Biophys Res Commun.* 1969; 36(5): 838–43.
7. Trivelli LA, Ranney HM, Lai HT. Hemoglobin components in patients with diabetes mellitus. *N Engl J Med.* 1971; 284(7): 353–7.
8. Bry L, Chen PC, Sacks DB. Effects of hemoglobin variants and chemically modified derivatives on assays for glycohemoglobin. *Clin Chem.* 2001; 47(2): 153–63.
9. Little RR, Rohlfing CL, Wiedmeyer HM, Myers GL, Sacks DB, Goldstein DE, et al. The national glycohemoglobin standardization program: a five-year progress report. *Clin Chem.* 2001; 47(11): 1985–92.
10. Shemin D, Rittenberg D. The life span of the human red blood cell. *J Biol Chem.* 1946; 166(2): 627–36.
11. Nathan DM, Singer DE, Hurxthal K, Goodson JD. The clinical information value of the glycosylated hemoglobin assay. *N Engl J Med.* 1984; 310(6): 341–6.
12. Gomez-Perez FJ, Aguilar-Salinas CA, Almeda-Valdes P, Cuevas-Ramos D, Lerman Garber I, Rull JA. HbA1c for the diagnosis of diabetes mellitus in a developing country. A position article. *Arch Med Res.* 2010; 41(4): 302–8.
13. Timar B, Albai O. The relationship between hemoglobin a1c and chronic complications in diabetes mellitus. *Rom J Diabetes Nutr Metab Dis.* 2012; 19(2): 115–22.
14. Waikato District Health Board. Laboratory test reference guide. www.waikatodhbgovtnz/lab/. 2012.
15. Control D, Group CTR. The effect of intensive treatment of diabetes on the development and progression of long-term complications in insulin-dependent diabetes mellitus. *N Engl J Med.* 1993; 329(14): 977–86.
16. Peter A, Fritsche A, Stefan N, Heni M, Haring HU, Schleicher E. Diagnostic value of hemoglobin A1c for type 2 diabetes mellitus in a population at risk. *Exp Clin Endocrinol Diabetes.* 2011; 119(4): 234–7.
17. Van'T Riet E, Alssema M, Rijkelijkhuizen JM, Kostense PJ, Nijpels G, Dekker JM. Relationship between A1C and glucose levels in the general Dutch population: the New Hoorn Study. *Diabetes Care.* 2010; 33(1): 61–6.

18. National Glycohemoglobin Standardization Program. Background. www.ngsporg/bgroundasp. 1996.

19. Jeppsson JO, Kobold U, Barr J, Finke A, Hoelzel W, Hoshino T, et al. Approved IFCC reference method for the measurement of HbA1c in human blood. *Clin Chem Lab Med*. 2002; 40(1): 78–89.

20. Finke A, Kobold U, Hoelzel W, Weykamp C, Miedema K, Jeppsson JO. Preparation of a candidate primary reference material for the international standardisation of HbA1c determinations. *Clin Chem Lab Med*. 1998; 36(5): 299–308.

21. Geistanger A, Arends S, Berding C, Hoshino T, Jeppsson JO, Little R, et al. Statistical methods for monitoring the relationship between the IFCC reference measurement procedure for hemoglobin A1c and the designated comparison methods in the United States, Japan, and Sweden. *Clin Chem*. 2008; 54(8): 1379–85.

22. Nathan DM, Kuenen J, Borg R, Zheng H, Schoenfeld D, Heine RJ, et al. Translating the A1C assay into estimated average glucose values. *Diabetes Care*. 2008; 31(8): 1473–8.

23. Sacks DB, Assay AEIWGotHc. Global harmonization of hemoglobin A1c. *Clin Chem*. 2005; 51(4): 681–3.

24. Hoelzel W, Weykamp C, Jeppsson JO, Miedema K, Barr JR, Goodall I, et al. IFCC reference system for measurement of hemoglobin A1c in human blood and the national standardization schemes in the United States, Japan, and Sweden: a method-comparison study. *Clin Chem*. 2004; 50(1): 166–74.

25. Hanas R, John WG, International Hb AcCC. 2013 update on the worldwide standardization of the HbA1c measurement. *Diabetes Med*. 2013; 30(7): 885–6.

26. Fleming JK. Evaluation of HbA1c on the Roche COBAS Integra 800 closed tube system. *Clin Biochem*. 2007; 40(11): 822–7.

27. Weykamp C, John WG, Mosca A. A review of the challenge in measuring hemoglobin A1c. *J Diabetes Sci Technol*. 2009; 3(3): 439–45.

28. HbA1c assay interferences. www.ngsporg/interfasp. 2015.

29. Goldenberg RM, Cheng AY, Punthakee Z, Clement M. Use of glycated hemoglobin (A1C) in the diagnosis of type 2 diabetes mellitus in adults. *Can J Diabetes*. 2011; 35(3): 247–9.

30. Virtue MA, Furne JK, Nuttall FQ, Levitt MD. Relationship between GHb concentration and erythrocyte survival determined from breath carbon monoxide concentration. *Diabetes Care*. 2004; 27(4): 931–5.

31. Vashist SK, Zheng D, Al-Rubeaan K, Luong JHT, Sheu FS. Technology behind commercial devices for blood glucose monitoring in diabetes management: a review. *Anal Chim Acta*. 2011; 703(2): 124–36.

32. Little RR, Lenters-Westra E, Rohlfing CL, Slingerland R. Point-of-care assays for hemoglobin A(1c): is performance adequate? *Clin Chem*. 2011; 57(9): 1333–4.

33. Leca V, Ibrahim Z, Lombard-Pontou E, Maraninchi M, Guieu R, Portugal H, et al. Point-of-care measurements of HbA(1c): simplicity does not mean laxity with controls. *Diabetes Care.* 2012; 35(12):e85.

34. Lenters-Westra E, Slingerland RJ. Hemoglobin A1c point-of-care assays; a new world with a lot of consequences! *J Diabetes Sci Technol.* 2009; 3(3): 418–23.

35. Lenters-Westra E, Slingerland RJ. Six of eight hemoglobin A1c point-of-care instruments do not meet the general accepted analytical performance criteria. *Clin Chem.* 2010; 56(1): 44–52.

36. Lenters-Westra E, Slingerland RJ. Evaluation of the Quo-Test hemoglobin A1c point-of-care instrument: second chance. *Clin Chem.* 2010; 56(7): 1191–3.

37. Lenters-Westra E, Slingerland RJ. Three of 7 hemoglobin A1c point-of-care instruments do not meet generally accepted analytical performance criteria. *Clin Chem.* 2014; 60(8): 1062–72.

38. Szymezak J, Leroy N, Lavalard E, Gillery P. Evaluation of the DCA Vantage analyzer for HbA1c assay. *Clin Chem Lab Med.* 2008; 46(8): 1195–8.

39. Sanchez-Mora C, M SR-O, Fernandez-Riejos P, Mateo J, Polo-Padillo J, Goberna R, et al. Evaluation of two HbA1c point-of-care analyzers. *Clin Chem Lab Med.* 2011; 49(4): 653–7.

40. Little RR, Roberts WL. A review of variant hemoglobins interfering with hemoglobin A1c measurement. *J Diabetes Sci Technol.* 2009; 3(3): 446–51.

41. Direct Enzymatic HbA1c assay. www.diazymecom/direct-enzymatic-hba1c. 2015.

42. Armbruster DA. Fructosamine: structure, analysis, and clinical usefulness. *Clin Chem.* 1987; 33(12): 2153–63.

43. Johnson RN, Metcalf PA, Baker JR. Fructosamine: a new approach to the estimation of serum glycosylprotein. An index of diabetic control. *Clin Chim Acta.* 1983; 127(1): 87–95.

44. Schleicher E, Wieland OH. Specific quantitation by HPLC of protein (lysine) bound glucose in human serum albumin and other glycosylated proteins. *J Clin Chem Clin Biochem.* 1981; 19(2): 81–7.

45. Schleicher E, Mayer R, Wagner EM, Gerbitz K-D. Is serum fructosamine assay specific for determination of glycated serum protein? *Clin Chem.* 1988; 34(2): 320–3.

46. Schleicher ED, Olgemoller B, Wiedenmann E, Gerbitz KD. Specific glycation of albumin depends on its half-life. *Clin Chem.* 1993; 39(4): 625–8.

47. Pundir CS, Chawla S. Determination of glycated hemoglobin with special emphasis on biosensing methods. *Anal Biochem.* 2014; 444:47–56.

48. Tominaga M, Makino H, Yoshino G, Kuwa K, Takei I, Aono Y, et al. Report of the Committee on Standardization of Laboratory Testing Related to Diabetes Mellitus of the Japan Diabetes Society: Determination of Reference Intervals Hemoglobin A1c (IFCC) and Glycoalbumin in Japanese Population. *J Japan Diabetes Soc.* 2006; 49(10): 825.

49. Paroni R, Ceriotti F, Galanello R, Battista Leoni G, Panico A, Scurati E, et al. Performance characteristics and clinical utility of an enzymatic method for the measurement of glycated albumin in plasma. *Clin Biochem.* 2007; 40(18): 1398–405.

50. Miyashita Y, Nishimura R, Morimoto A, Matsudaira T, Sano H, Tajima N. Glycated albumin is low in obese, type 2 diabetic patients. *Diabetes Res Clin Pract.* 2007; 78(1): 51–5.

51. Koga M, Otsuki M, Matsumoto S, Saito H, Mukai M, Kasayama S. Negative association of obesity and its related chronic inflammation with serum glycated albumin but not glycated hemoglobin levels. *Clin Chim Acta.* 2007; 378(1): 48–52.

52. Koga M, Murai J, Saito H, Matsumoto S, Kasayama S. Effects of thyroid hormone on serum glycated albumin levels: study on non-diabetic subjects. *Diabetes Res Clin Pract.* 2009; 84(2): 163–7.

CHAPTER 6

Diabetes management software and smart applications

Sandeep Kumar Vashist and John HT Luong

CHAPTER SUMMARY

There has been continuous improvement in diabetes management software during the last decade, resulting in much better management of diabetes with easy analysis, trend prediction, better data visualisation, and safe and secure data storage. Although most of the efforts in this direction have been devoted by the industrial giants that hold a significant market share of glucose monitoring devices, some of the software has also been developed by other companies. The recent years have seen a tremendous rise in the number of cellphone users, crossing the 7 billion mark and now present in 98% of the world population. The emergence of smartphone-based glucose monitoring devices and healthcare applications has further led to the development of several prospective smart applications for diabetic glucose monitoring and management. With the advent of Cloud computing and wearable smart gadgets such as smart watches, these smart applications are providing an effective universal platform for diabetic management with improved mobile health and telemedicine tools.

Keywords: diabetes management; software; smart applications; glucose monitoring.

CONTENTS

INTRODUCTION

The management of diabetes is of immense value as it is the only way that diabetics can have a normal lifestyle, avoiding costly and lethal diabetic complications. However, it is widely known that in today's world where the number of doctors is much fewer than the number of diabetics worldwide, the management of diabetes can only be done effectively by empowering diabetics with skills, knowledge, tools and technologies that will motivate them to take charge of their health. The big industrial giants that account for the predominant share of the home glucose monitoring market have invested intensive efforts to develop highly effective and truly advanced diabetic management software that enable glucose monitoring data, which is easy to read and analyse and has trend prediction and data history. These include ACCU-CHEK® 360° diabetes management system by Roche,[1] FreeStyle CoPilot health management system by Abbott,[2] CareLink® personal therapy management software by Medtronic,[3] Dexcom STUDIO software by Dexcom,[4] and OneTouch® diabetes management software by LifeScan.[5]

The last few years have seen a revolutionary change in mobile healthcare with many new smartphones and smart wearable gadget-based mH devices already penetrating the market and being used by millions of diabetics worldwide. Presently, mH has transformed into a major healthcare delivery concept for all healthcare and bioanalytical settings. The mH market is estimated to reach US$26 billion by 2017.[6] The development of the world's smallest FDA-approved and

CE-certified smartphone-based blood glucose meter, iHealth Align,[7] is a breakthrough in diabetes management. Smartphones have become ubiquitous and are the ideal point-of-care device for mobile health-care.[8-11] A large number of smart applications have been developed for diabetics for the monitoring of glucose and other basic physiological parameters. However, despite having more than 1100 smart applications for diabetes,[12] GluCoMo™ by Artificial Life, Inc.[13] and iHealth Gluco-Smart[14] by iHealth Labs are the most prominent smart applications for diabetic glucose monitoring and management. Apart from providing educational modules and tips to diabetics about effective management of diabetes, these smart applications have placed tremendous power in the hands of diabetics. They are equipped with all essential features that enable the diabetic to live a healthy lifestyle without spending a lot of time on the meticulous planning of numerous tasks that they have to follow routinely. Therefore, it has significantly increased the compliance of diabetics and led to better health outcomes with critically reduced healthcare costs pertaining to diabetes management, which drain most of the healthcare expenditure worldwide. The smart applications-based self-management of diabetes empowers the diabetics and makes them aware of the need for a lifestyle change and adopting a healthy lifestyle, resulting in reduced diabetic complications.[15-17] The American Diabetes Association has further recommended the integration of data and information from the self-monitoring of blood glucose into clinical and self-management plans.[17]

The emerging trend is towards the smart gadget-based wearable healthcare technologies such as smart watches that monitor the basic physiological parameters like physical activity and pulse in real time. The coming years will witness many of the diabetic blood glucose monitoring devices and smart applications for diabetic management being successfully adapted to smart watches. iHealth Gluco-Smart has already been adapted to be used in the smart watch.

This chapter describes the main characteristics and features of the various commercially available diabetic management software and smart applications along with the emerging challenges of big data and mH, and their prospects.

DIABETES MANAGEMENT SOFTWARE
ACCU-CHEK® 360° diabetes management system

The ACCU-CHEK® 360° diabetes management system[1] is PC-based software developed by Roche.[1] It provides a collection of all the glucose measurement readings from the glucose meters provided by Roche securely into the software. It offers highly simplified visualisation of the results in the form of easy-to-read but comprehensive graphs, which enables diabetics to take timely action in order to improve their diabetic management. The users can customise the reports based on their personalised needs and create express reports instantaneously. The blood glucose meter measurements and the insulin pump information can be downloaded and integrated on a single graph, thereby providing more detailed information about diabetes management. Moreover, it also enables diabetics to visualise the effects of nutritional, dietary, physical activity and other lifestyle interventions, and/or medications, on the blood glucose readings by analysing the trend. The customisable reports are an added advantage to diabetic healthcare professionals as they provide them with very useful information about patients, leading to a more effective treatment plan. The software is compatible with ACCU-CHEK Aviva Expert meter, ACCU-CHEK Aviva Combo meter, ACCU-CHEK Spirit Combo insulin pump, and ACCU-CHEK Spirit insulin pump.

FreeStyle CoPilot health management system

The FreeStyle CoPilot health management system[2] has been developed by Abbott as a versatile data management tool that allows diabetics, caregivers and healthcare professionals to manage diabetes effectively, taking into consideration the informed insights provided by the software reports. The software interfaces with the supported blood glucose monitoring devices from Abbott Diabetes Care, which enables it to upload the recorded glucose test results into the software for comprehensive analysis and interpretation. The users record useful information about medication, meals, carbohydrate intake, exercise, physical activities, insulin, ketones, medical exams, lab results and general notes. Similar to other software, it also displays glucose trends and patterns together with the insulin dosage and carbohydrate intake. It provides easy-to-read visual graphs, charts and reports that enable much better analysis of blood glucose readings and diabetic health management plans. The reports can be printed and sent to a healthcare provider or other persons. The software provides 12 reports for the glucose readings, consisting of diary list, glucose modal day, glucose line, glucose average, glucose histogram, glucose pie chart, logbook, lab and exam record, statistics, daily combination view, weekly pump view and healthcare professional group analysis. Further, the software provides a 2-week glucose summary with logbook report, which provides a consolidated view of glucose modal day, glucose pie, statistics and logbook reports for the specified 2 weeks. The glucose modal day report shows the daily pattern of glucose levels while the glucose line report provides a visualisation of trends in glucose levels. The glucose average report shows the blood glucose averages pre- and post-meal times of the day, which helps in identifying the specific times of the day that require more glucose testing or control. The glucose histogram and pie chart reports provide concise histogram and pie chart views, respectively, of all glucose readings into the default target zones. The logbook report is a tabular depiction of glucose readings, carbohydrate intake and insulin doses taken during the day. The lab and exam record report provides a table containing data from all lab tests and medical exams during the specified period. The statistics provide pre- and post-meal glucose readings, carbohydrate intake and insulin dosages taken over the specified date range in a tabular format. The glucose statistics table provides glucose readings in a day together with the highest and lowest readings in each time period with average glucose and standard deviations within and across various time periods. The insulin statistics provide a tabular depiction of average insulin dosages over the specified date range. If insulin is being administered by the diabetic using an insulin pump, the pump statistics report will provide the insulin pump statistics instead of the insulin statistics. The healthcare professional group analysis report is exclusively available to the healthcare professionals to view the data for all the patients being managed by them.

The software has two modes: Home User for diabetics and HCP for healthcare professionals. Each diabetic and healthcare professional has a unique profile that is protected by a secure password. The software allows multiple home users, members of a family, and multiple healthcare professionals, in a clinic and hospital, to share the use of the software. The users can share their data and recorded health information with their healthcare professionals by synchronising them via the Internet.

CareLink® personal therapy management software

CareLink® personal therapy management software[3] has been developed by Medtronic for the gathering and analysis of glucose measurement and insulin delivery data from Medtronic glucose meters, continuous glucose monitoring systems, and Medtronic insulin pumps. It enables the user to determine precisely insulin intake based on the glucose levels in addition to analysing the effect on glucose levels of physical activity and meals. The software acts as a virtual logbook, which enables the user to plot charts and graphs for easy-to-read data analysis and visualisation. The actual data are still stored in the form of tables. The CareLink® data analysis and reports enable the healthcare provider and the diabetic to discern glucose patterns easily in the data, and the associated problems, so that the provider can rapidly and precisely make appropriate adjustments in the therapy. Moreover, it enables the healthcare provider to access remotely and review the CareLink® data of the diabetic patient, which provides critical insights into the glucose patterns. The visualisation of glucose patterns enables the diabetic to prevent dangerous hypogly-caemic episodes during the night to maintain strict control of glucose levels within the euglycaemic range. Moreover, it also provides them with the effects of certain foods and their portion sizes on their blood glucose levels, thereby enabling better diabetes management. The beneficial effects of using the CareLink® personal software for diabetic management has been demonstrated by a study that has shown that the software users have improved control of glycated haemoglobin (HbA1c), which is an indicator of long-term average of blood glucose levels, in comparison to diabetics that employed only insulin pump therapy without any software.[18]

Dexcom STUDIO software

Dexcom STUDIO[4] is the diabetes management software developed by Dexcom that interfaces with Dexcom glucose meters, such as Dexcom G4 Platinum continuous glucose monitor, and downloads the glu-cose measurement data. The software provides glucose distribution, glucose trends, hourly statistics, daily statistics and daily trends along with the Success Report and Dexcom PORTRAIT summary report. The Dexcom PORTRAIT summary report is a one-page report that provides an immediate analysis and statistics of the important bio-analytical parameters pertaining to diabetic glucose management. The report enables identification of the clinically significant patterns and prioritisation of particular glucose patterns to be addressed with the pattern map. It also identifies the most significant patterns to be targeted along with an insightful summary. Moreover, it provides the strategies that can be employed for better diabetic glucose manage-ment with possible considerations and interpretation. The pattern map provides an easy-to-read visual graph about the clinically signifi-cant glycaemic excursions, such as night-time and daytime highs and lows, along with possible considerations to avoid such excursions. Additionally, it highlights the most significant hyper- and hypo-glycaemic excursions together with their frequency of occurrence. Moreover, it provides a summary of glucose statistics and calibration frequency along with therapy considerations and suggestions for better glycaemic control. The hourly and daily statistics reports provide an assessment of the hourly and daily glycaemic patterns together with the variability, while the trends reports provide an assessment of glycaemic patterns. The glucose distribution report shows the percentage time of high, low and in target glucose ranges together with the overall glucose distribution and assessment of pre- and postprandial control. Moreover, the success report provides glycaemic control weekly, monthly or quarterly, which enables diabetics to keep track of their glycaemic control and motivates them to achieve and sustain tight glycaemic control for improved diabetes management. However, Dexcom STUDIO is only available on Windows operating systems. Dexcom provides another similar software, Dexcom CLARITY™, for Mac users, which has the same features, along with Dexcom Clarity's Dashboard to provide all the essential information and the most relevant insights for diabetes blood glucose management.

OneTouch® diabetes management software

OneTouch® diabetes management software[5] is developed by LifeScan for the efficient management of glucose measurement data, which can be obtained using the data port of any of the more than 15 OneTouch® blood glucose meters that have been developed by LifeScan. It provides an easy-to-read and comprehensive visual picture of the glucose measurement data along with 11 powerful reports that can easily identify glucose trends, such as night-time and daytime highs and lows together with the best daytime and meal-related patterns daily, weekly, monthly or quarterly. The 11 reports provided by the software are the logbook, 14-day summary, glucose trend, pie chart, average reading, standard day, data list, histogram, insulin, exception and health checks. The reports provide an analysis of the glucose results taking into consideration the factors that affect them and highlighting the out-of-target range results. They can be viewed by users and shared with healthcare providers. The software enables the addition of information to a patient record apart from enabling the addition or editing of information for a glucose measurement. The logbook report provides information on glucose levels and trends along with an analysis of health-related data that can impact the readings. The pie chart report gives the percentage of glucose measurements that are within, above and below the specific target range. The glucose trend report provides analysis of track changes in glucose readings from one day to another. The 14-day summary report provides a graphical summary of the logbook, pie chart and glucose trend reports for a particular 14-day period. The standard day report identifies the pattern in the glucose measurements by the time of day. The histogram report enables the identification of pre- and post-meal patterns in glucose values, while the average reading report monitors the average glucose measurements and determines the impact of exercise, physical activities and meals on the average glucose value. The data list report provides a sequential view of all data in the software data such as glucose, exercise, physical activities and medications. The exception report ranks the patients on the basis of key diabetic glucose management measures and screens out those that require closer management. The insulin report provides an analysis of the relation between glucose levels, carbohydrate intake in meals, and the insulin doses. Additionally, the health checks report provides an analysis of the effects of diabetes on other health factors such as blood pressure, weight, HbA1c level and doctor visits. The reports can be printed, faxed or shared with another person or healthcare provider. Moreover, the information can be added to the patient record.

SMART APPLICATIONS
iHealth Gluco-Smart

iHealth Gluco-Smart[14] (Fig. 6.1) is a smart application developed by iHealth Labs Inc. that works with the iHealth Gluco-Monitoring System or iHealth Align. iHealth Gluco-Monitoring System is interfaced to the iOS and Android operating system-based smartphones by low energy Bluetooth transfer. In contrast, iHealth Align is a next-generation smartphone-based blood glucose meter that plugs in directly to the 3.5 mm audio jack of the smartphone and transfers data in real time to the iHealth Gluco-Smart. The smart application critically reduces the handling time by automatic and smart handling of all glucose monitoring tasks, which include the logging of glucose test results, coding, and counting of the test strips. The digital logbook of test results eliminates errors due to manual entry. The glucose test results are saved securely to the free and personalised iHealth Cloud service, where the diabetic is required to set up his/her account. It enables the easy analysis and visualisation of glucose test results anywhere and at any place where Internet or Wi-Fi are available. The smart application is equipped with four major features of measure, record, manage and share. The measuring mode enables the user to view the glucose test results in real time on the smartphone, which can then be supplemented and tagged with further details such as physical activities, meals taken and voice memo. It also uploads the

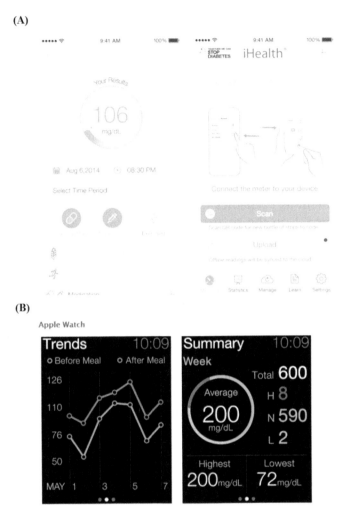

FIGURE 6.1 iHealth Gluco-Smart. Screenshots of the smart application on (A) iPhone, and (B) Apple Watch. Images are copyright of iHealth Labs Inc. (Reproduced with permission from iHealth Labs Inc.)

offline glucose test measurements and scans the new test strips that enable smart tracking. The record mode provides an easy-to-read graphical summary of glucose measurements and averages of a user for up to the past 3 months, where the readings are stored securely in the iHealth Cloud account of the user. The managing mode provides a review of the personal digital logbook that contains all the comprehensive details of the glucose measurements: the time and date stamp when the reading was taken together with the meals, carbohydrates, physical activity and voice memo of the user. It also enables the user to visualise the trends and the statistics of the glucose measurements during the day, which motivates the user to effectively manage the hypo- or hyperglycaemic episodes during the specific times predicted by the trend glucose curve. Additionally, the user can set up alarm alerts and reminders to take glucose measurements, insulin and/or other medication for more effective diabetes management. The company has also developed a smart application for the Apple Watch, which enables users to view their past week's glucose measurement data with trends and statistics without any need for opening the smart application automatically. Moreover, it enables even better diabetes management as it enables the user to receive notifications for the reminders set on the smartphone. Additionally, the company has developed a dedicated smart application for healthcare professionals, iHealth Pro, which has all the functions of iHealth Gluco-Smart but further enables healthcare providers to visualise the data pertaining to unlimited patient profiles.

GluCoMo™

GluCoMo™[13] is a smart application developed by Artificial Life, Inc. (Fig. 6.2) for the management of diabetic monitoring and patient coaching. The smart application is available for purchase at iTunes store at a nominal price of US$0.99. It has well-developed telematics features compatible with various platforms, such as iOS, Android, Symbian, Windows Phone 7 and Java. The application is very useful for diabetics as it allows them to monitor and accordingly manage their blood glucose levels, diet, insulin intake, physical activities, and basic physiological parameters such as blood pressure, pulse and weight. Therefore, it acts as an electronic diary and a reminder system for diabetics. The application has customised mobile client applications, an interactive web portal, and a secure telematics platform, which enables the data and information to be transferred to patients, doctors, hospitals, administrators and other authorised healthcare professionals. The 3G, 4G or Wi-Fi networks keep the data updated via the client application on a central database that can be accessed by certified doctors and authorised healthcare professionals only. It facilitates real-time communication between doctors and patients and also inter-hospital communication, where doctors can share advice, and provide medical opinions and diagnostics directly to the patient. Moreover, it issues warnings to the diabetics in case dangerous trends are detected in their glucose readings and advises them to keep the blood glucose under control by pursuing the desired physical

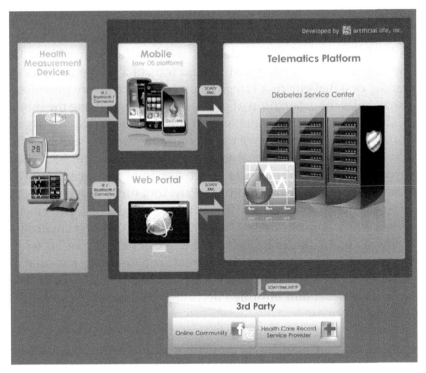

FIGURE 6.2 GluCoMo™ developed by Artificial Life, Inc. (Reproduced with permission from Artificial Life, Inc.)

activities. The smart application employs various methods for data encryption, such as secure authentication, firewall, anti-virus, secure data transport and data storage, thereby enabling effective data management. It enables diabetics to set up alarmed automated alerts to remind them of engaging in various physical activities after reviewing their entry history in the graph, thereby providing an effective lifestyle intervention. Moreover, the diabetics can also engage in online interactions and sharing via built-in forums, and have continued access to an informative diabetes handbook that acts as an educational tool to acquire diabetic facts, prevalence, monitoring and management.

ACCU-CHEK® Connect and Glooko™ app

ACCU-CHEK® Connect diabetes management app[19] is a smart application developed by Roche that is compatible with Apple and Android smart devices, having Bluetooth® Smart technology. The application can be linked with ACCU-CHEK Aviva Connect meter and receives the glucose readings data wirelessly by Bluetooth® Smart technology. It requires the users to create their personal ACCU-CHEK Connect online portal account, which enables them to review and visualise the glucose measurements data, generate reports, and share the data and information with their doctors and healthcare providers. The application can be customised to send texts of a new blood glucose reading of a diabetic to a caregiver, parent or healthcare provider. It also enables the calculation of precise insulin doses using the inbuilt ACCU-CHEK Bolus Advisor[20] within the app after activation by the doctor, which makes it easy to determine mealtime insulin. It has a 3-day profile tool that enables visualisation of the glucose trends curve and analyses the effects of activity, food and insulin on the blood glucose levels. The Testing in Paris tool further determines the effect of meals, stress or activity on the blood glucose. The glucose measurement data received by the ACCU-CHEK® Connect application is stored automatically in the Cloud and can be accessed anywhere by ACCU-CHEK Connect online portal. The extensive information provides highly useful information and data to the doctors, thereby facilitating better and informed decisions that lead to improved diabetic management.

Glooko™ app[21] is a smart application developed by Roche for diabetic management. It is compatible with iPhone and Android-based smartphones, and can collect and view diabetes data from any ACCU-CHEK blood glucose meter. The ACCU-CHEK Aviva Connect meter connects to the Glooko™ app after automatic synchronisation of blood glucose readings, while a Glooko MeterSync Blue device is required to upload glucose measurement data from other ACCU-CHEK meters. It enables the user to add pre- and post-meal notes about the carbohydrate intake, activity, and/or insulin doses and visualise their effect on the blood glucose profile. Moreover, the built-in database of more than 200,000 foods enables better determination of glucose values, thereby facilitating more precise insulin dosing. Similar to the other smart application, it also provides easy-to-read track trends in glucose readings and the analysis of data, which motivates diabetics to manage their blood glucose level by lifestyle, nutritional or medical intervention. The users can also set up reminders with push notifications on a smartphone for blood glucose measurements, insulin injections or taking medication. Moreover, they can share their data and reports with their healthcare providers and additionally use Glooko ProConnect to share data with other websites or online dashboards.

CHALLENGES

Diabetes management software and smart applications are empowering diabetics to become active decision makers, which is paving the way to better healthcare monitoring and management. It is leading to critically improved and sustained health outcomes as well as reducing healthcare costs. Moreover, the quality of the enriched data, which can be accessed anywhere by patients and doctors and at any time, is leading to improved strategies for healthcare delivery in real time by employing the tools for telemedicine and communication that are already integrated within such software and smart applications. These developments have shown the successful convergence of various scientific disciplines, such as engineering, bioanalytical sciences, biomedicine and physical sciences, to develop innovative technologies for mH. The ongoing research in smart systems and technologies together with increased functionalities and tools for mH and telemedicine in software will further lead to highly sophisticated next-generation smart applications for personalised diabetic monitoring and management. These smart applications will enable diabetics to analyse their blood glucose readings and adjust their lifestyle accordingly to achieve improved and sustained health benefits. Moreover, they will improve the patients' knowledge, behaviour and efficiency that would enable more effective diabetes management.[22]

The continuous developments in mH and telemedicine together with the significant increase in funding and a rapid growth in public interest for improved healthcare and better health management tools are facilitating the development of novel smart applications for diabetes management. The most recent FDA clearance and CE accreditation of iHealth Align, the world's smallest smartphone-based blood glucose meter, is a remarkable advance, which will inspire the development of novel diabetic monitoring devices. Current efforts focus on overcoming the technical challenges such as rapidly evolving models of smartphones, data security and storage, compliance with bioanalytical and regulatory guidelines, and achieving the high analytical performance criteria as desired for POC devices.

The described commercial diabetic management software and smart applications are already being used by millions of diabetics worldwide, who have reported highly simplified diabetic monitoring and management, better compliance, decreased hyperglycaemic and hypoglycaemic episodes, and improved health outcomes. It has significantly reduced the number of visits of diabetics to doctors and prevented diabetic complications, thereby resulting in significant cost savings by frequent glucose testing and simple physical activity, lifestyle and/or nutritional interventions. The recent mH devices and continuously increasing trend towards the development of mH can be revolutionised by providing gigantic data via centralised Cloud computing, to establish enriched information for more predictive healthcare monitoring and management in societies.

The recent developments in Cloud computing in the last few years are providing the impetus for rapidly increasing mH applications, leading to improved healthcare delivery and significant cost savings by reduced infrastructure and operational costs.[23] However, it has also given rise to growing concerns about data security and privacy of personal information.[24-26] The national laws and guidelines of most countries have stressed the need for physically storing the data within the national boundaries, which requires substantial research and development efforts that will enable Cloud computing to comply with these stringent norms.[27] This limitation has been counteracted successfully by Amazon and Google. The Government Cloud product from Google allows countries to store data as per their national data security guidelines. Similarly, Amazon Web Services also permits businesses to store data within their national boundaries. Considering the enormous developments in Cloud computing, there is a growing need for the creation of international Cloud computing standards. This has resulted in several initiatives, such as EuroCloud and Google's Data Liberation Front, with the primary focus on establishing international standards. Moreover, the protection of the privacy of personal information data in personal electronic health records (PEHRs) is the most sensitive and challenging issue of potential concern. International ethical guidelines clearly state that patients have complete ownership and should have complete control of their PEHRs. But there is a need for clear guidelines stating the ownership of the data pertaining to medical information and the responsibility to safeguard private information.[28] Therefore, the sensitive personal information of patients should never be exposed to third-party servers and unauthorised parties. At the moment, this concern is being addressed by implementing attribute-based encryption[29] strategies, engaging an authorised and trusted third party,[27] and employing advanced Cloud computing models that ensure security and privacy of personal data.[30] However, the information security on the Cloud is highly robust and in fact much better than the security strategies employed by government agencies and leading companies.[31,32] The benefit of employing PEHRs is well known to healthcare professionals, the community and patients as it leads to critical improvements in caregivers' decisions and patients' health outcomes.[33] This has resulted in the establishment of the Health Information Technology for Economic and Clinical Health Act (HITECH) in the United States, which offers authorised incentive payments through insurance agencies to the healthcare practitioners, who use PEHRs to achieve specified improvements in healthcare delivery.[34] The developed diabetic smart applications employ smartphone-based mobile Cloud computing,[35] which is providing next-generation mH technology for personalised healthcare monitoring and management.[36]

Presently, most of the diabetic smart applications are driven by the market push without major clinical or pilot studies, where the role of the healthcare provider is either negligible or missing. Moreover, most of these do not provide the functionalities for intelligent coaching and behavioural management. This substantiates the need for more robust, systematic, regulated and clinically validated smart applications in the near future for centralised diabetes management with more functionalities. Moreover, many diabetic smart applications also need careful evaluation and patients should be informed about trusted applications and their utility.[37] The United States FDA has recently issued guidelines and procedures for the regulation of various mobile medical applications, including those for diabetes management.[38] Similarly, the guidelines are being revised by the European Union for the regulation of smart applications for healthcare, which fall under the EU medical devices directive 93/42/EEC.[39] However, there are many open challenges, such as ethical issues, personal privacy issues, data ownership, data processing in open platforms, and efficacy and regulatory perspective, which will be tackled effectively with focused and intensive efforts in the coming years.

A recent survey identifies the major frustrations that the diabetics experience daily pertaining to their diabetes monitoring and management.[40] Diabetics require daily care and more frequent visits to their healthcare providers. Most of the diabetics acknowledge the fact that they need to be empowered and engaged to manage their health. Moreover, they know the importance of keeping their blood glucose level controlled by frequent testing and lifestyle interventions. However, diabetics' major frustrations are a lack of interaction with healthcare providers, difficulties in scheduling appointments, lack of timely communications with healthcare providers, and challenges in managing the complex care of diabetes. Based on the survey, a set of recommendations has been provided for more effective diabetes care and management. There is a need for centralised real-time access, which can be achieved by making patients' medical records readily available and accessible to all healthcare providers of the patients via a nationwide PEHR system. There is also a need for timely electronic access to expected and completed laboratory work, which can be implemented if each healthcare provider adopts an online reservation system. This will enable diabetics to schedule their appointments and get confirmations and reminders as well as laboratory results. Quest Diagnostics has developed such a smart application-based system called MyQuest.[41] Obviously, if patients have access to their laboratory results, they are more aware of their health and ask much better questions.[42] Similarly, an online scheduling system should be implemented, which will enable the patients to search the healthcare providers in their area and submit an appointment reservation request. A similar system has been demonstrated by ZocDoc.[43] The last recommendation was the need for tools for better management of diabetes, such as glucose monitoring and medication reminders; alerts for low insulin volume in the insulin pump and need to check the blood glucose level manually; text messaging from healthcare team members; and intelligent and interactive PEHR systems. A recent study has shown that text messaging to poorly controlled diabetic adults was very useful to encourage the patients, which showed improved glycaemic control.[44] The text message can be customised to provide a personalised treatment plan and advice, taking into account the need and preferences of the patients.

The cost and reimbursement also play a prominent role as most insurance plans do not cover the diabetic management software, smart applications and educational programmes that are desired for mH.[45] The healthcare providers need to be provided with mH-equipped software and smart applications together with interactive web-based learning tools[46] to manage the health of their registered diabetics. However, online social networking services have to be used with care in diabetes management,[47] taking into account the enormous risk and challenge concerning the authenticity of the information provided and the provider.

The continuously increasing features and capabilities of smartphones and smart wearable gadgets together with the evolving next-generation mobile Cloud computing and contributing technologies will lead to highly innovative smart applications and software for effective diabetic management that will be more clinically acceptable. The upcoming operating systems in such smart devices will have truly advanced features apart from fitness, health tracking, GPRS tracking, and dedicated Healthbook application. Moreover, such devices will be offered at an affordable cost due to the rapidly increasing number of users in developed as well as developing nations.

CONCLUSIONS

Diabetes management software and smart applications are playing a prominent role in empowering diabetics to manage their health effectively by continuous tracking of their blood glucose and keeping it sustained within the normal physiological range. They are equipped with easy analysis and better visualisation of glucose-sensing data apart from predicting the trend in glucose and setting up of automated alarmed alerts and reminders. The automated alarmed alerts enable diabetics to control their glucose level if it goes outside the normal range. Moreover, diabetics can set up automated reminders to monitor their blood glucose levels more frequently including when engaging in physical activities, thereby maintaining an active and healthy lifestyle. The upcoming trend of wearable gadgets such as smart watches is further providing a fully integrated healthcare solution as they will continuously monitor the physical activity and basic physiological parameters of users, which will enable them to manage their diabetes via the data, alerts and reminders issued by the smart application.

REFERENCES

1. ACCU-CHEK® 360° diabetes management system. www.accu-chekcom/us/data-management/360-softwarehtml. 2016.
2. FreeStyle CoPilot Health Management System. www.myfreestylecom/copilot-software. 2016.
3. CareLink® Personal Therapy Management Software. www.medtronic diabetescom/products/carelink-personal-diabetes-software. 2016.
4. Dexcom Studio. www.dexcomcom/dexcom-studio. 2016.
5. OneTouch® Diabetes Management Software. www.onetouchcom/software_kit. 2016.
6. 1.7B to download health apps by 2017. http://mobihealthnewscom/20814/report-1-7b-to-download-health-apps-by-2017. 2016.
7. iHealth Align. https://ihealthlabscom/glucometer/ihealth-align/. 2016.
8. Kwon L, Long KD, Wan Y, Yu H, Cunningham BT. Medical diagnostics with mobile devices: comparison of intrinsic and extrinsic sensing. *Biotechnol Adv.* 2016; 34(3): 291–304.
9. Vashist SK, Luppa PB, Yeo LY, Ozcan A, Luong JHT. Emerging technologies for next-generation point-of-care testing. *Trends Biotechnol.* 2015; 33(11): 692–705.
10. Vashist SK, Mudanyali O, Schneider EM, Zengerle R, Ozcan A. Cellphone-based devices for bioanalytical sciences. *Anal Bioanal Chem.* 2014; 406(14): 3263–77.
11. Vashist SK, Schneider EM, Luong JHT. Commercial smartphone-based

devices and smart applications for personalized healthcare monitoring and management. *Diagnostics*. 2014; 4(3): 104–28.

12. Diabetes app market: how to leverage the full potential of the diabetes app market. https://research2guidancecom/wp-content/uploads/2015/08/Diabetes-App-Market-Report-2014-Previewpdf. 2016.

13. GluCoMo™. www.artificial-lifecom/en/products/mobile_content/business_apps/glucomo. 2016.

14. iHealth Gluco-Smart. https://ihealthlabscom/mobile-apps/. 2016.

15. Eng DS, Lee JM. The promise and peril of mobile health applications for diabetes and endocrinology. *Pediatr Diabetes*. 2013; 14(4): 231–8.

16. Schütt M, Kern W, Krause U, Busch P, Dapp A, Grziwotz R, et al. Is the frequency of self-monitoring of blood glucose related to long-term metabolic control? Multicenter analysis including 24,500 patients from 191 centers in Germany and Austria. *Exp Clin Endocrinol Diabetes*. 2006; 114(7): 384–8.

17. American Diabetes Association. Standards of medical care in diabetes – 2015. *Diabetes Care*. 2015; 38: S33–S40.

18. Corriveau EA, Durso PJ, Kaufman ED, Skipper BJ, Laskaratos LA, Heintzman KB. Effect of Carelink, an internet-based insulin pump monitoring system, on glycemic control in rural and urban children with type 1 diabetes mellitus. *Pediatr Diabetes*. 2008; 9(4 Pt 2): 360–6.

19. ACCU-CHEK® Connect diabetes management app. https://accu-chekcom/microsites/connect/. 2016.

20. Barnard K, Parkin C, Young A, Ashraf M. Use of an automated bolus calculator reduces fear of hypoglycemia and improves confidence in dosage accuracy in patients with type 1 diabetes mellitus treated with multiple daily insulin injections. *J Diabetes Sci Tech*. 2012; 6(1): 144–9.

21. Glooko™ app. www.accu-chekcom/us/data-management/glookohtml. 2016.

22. Guo SH-M, Chang H-K, Lin C-Y. Impact of mobile diabetes self-care system on patients' knowledge, behavior and efficacy. *Computers in Industry*. 2015; 69: 22–9.

23. Marston S, Li Z, Bandyopadhyay S, Zhang J, Ghalsasi A. Cloud computing: the business perspective. *Decision Support Systems*. 2011; 51(1): 176–89.

24. Subashini S, Kavitha V. A survey on security issues in service delivery models of cloud computing. *Journal of Network and Computer Applications*. 2011; 34(1): 1–11.

25. Sun D, Chang G, Sun L, Wang X. Surveying and analyzing security, privacy and trust issues in cloud computing environments. *Procedia Engineering*. 2011; 15: 2852–6.

26. Istepanian RS. Mobile applications for diabetes management: efficacy issues and regulatory challenges. *Lancet Diabetes Endocrinol*. 2015; 3(12): 921–3.

27. Zissis D, Lekkas D. Addressing cloud computing security issues. *Future Gener Comput Syst*. 2012; 28(3): 583–92.

28. Khansa L, Cook DF, James T, Bruyaka O. Impact of HIPAA provisions on the stock market value of healthcare institutions, and information security and other information technology firms. *Computers and Security*. 2012; 31(6): 750–70.

29. Li M, Yu S, Zheng Y, Ren K, Lou W. Scalable and secure sharing of personal health records in cloud computing using attribute-based encryption. *IEEE Transactions on Parallel and Distributed Systems*. 2013; 24(1): 131–43.

30. Schweitzer EJ. Reconciliation of the cloud computing model with US federal electronic health record regulations. *J Am Med Inform Assoc*. 2012; 19(2): 161–5.

31. Khansa L, Zobel CW. Assessing innovations in cloud security. *Journal of Computer Information Systems*. 2014; 54(3): 45–56.

32. Khansa L, Zobel CW, Goicochea G. Creating a taxonomy for mobile commerce innovations using social network and cluster analyses. *International Journal of Electronic Commerce*. 2012; 16(4): 19–52.

33. Blumenthal D, Tavenner M. The 'meaningful use' regulation for electronic health records. *New Engl J Med*. 2010; 363(6): 501–4.

34. Blumenthal D. Launching HITECH. *N Engl J Med*. 2010; 362(5): 382–5.

35. Dinh HT, Lee C, Niyato D, Wang P. A survey of mobile cloud computing: architecture, applications, and approaches. *Wireless Communications and Mobile Computing*. 2013; 13(18): 1587–611.

36. Boulos MN, Wheeler S, Tavares C, Jones R. How smartphones are changing the face of mobile and participatory healthcare: an overview, with example from eCAALYX. *Biomedical Engineering Online*. 2011; 10(1): 24.

37. Basilico A, Marceglia S, Bonacina S, Pinciroli F. Advising patients on selecting trustful apps for diabetes self-care. *Comput Biol Med*. 2016; 71: 86–96.

38. Administration UFaD. Mobile medical applications: guidance for industry and Food and Drug Administration staff. www.fdagov/downloads/MedicalDevices//UCM263366pdf. 2015.

39. Commission E. Revisions of medical device directives. http://eceuropaeu/growth/sectors/medical-devices/regulatory-framework/revision/index_enhtm. 2016.

40. Khansa L, Davis Z, Davis H, Chin A, Irvine H, Nichols L, et al. Health information technologies for patients with diabetes. *Technology in Society*. 2016; 44: 1–9.

41. Get Your Results On Your Mobile Phone. www.questdiagnosticscom/home/patients/get-results/mobile. 2015.

42. HHS strengthens patients' right to access lab test reports. www.hhsgov/about/news/2014/02/03/hhs-strengthens-patients-right-to-access-lab-test-reportshtml. 2014.

43. ZocDoc. www.zocdoc.com/. 2016.

44. Dobson R CK, Cutfield R, Hulme A, Hulme R, McNamara C, Maddison R, Murphy R, Shepherd M, Strydom J, Whittaker R. Diabetes Text-Message

Self-Management Support Program (SMS4BG): a pilot study. *JMIR mHealth uHealth*. 2015; 3(1):e32.

45. Practice transformation for physicians and health care teams. http://ndepnih gov/hcp-businesses-and-schools/practice-transformation/. 2016.

46. Rider BB, Lier SC, Johnson TK, Hu DJ. Interactive web-based learning: translating health policy into improved diabetes care. *Am J Prev Med*. 2016; 50(1): 122–8.

47. Toma T, Athanasiou T, Harling L, Darzi A, Ashrafian H. Online social networking services in the management of patients with diabetes mellitus: systematic review and meta-analysis of randomised controlled trials. *Diabetes Res Clin Pract*. 2014; 106(2): 200–11.

CHAPTER 7

Performance requirements, analytical accuracy and clinical accuracy of self-monitoring of blood glucose: a clinical perspective

Albert Donald Luong, Sandeep Kumar Vashist,
John HT Luong

CHAPTER SUMMARY

The accuracy of self-monitoring of blood glucose (SMBG) levels is the line of defence in diabetic control and management and plays an important role in the treatment and outcome of diabetes therapy. Also, point-of-care blood glucose monitoring is extended to rapid detection of extreme blood glucose concentrations in patients, who are in a coma or have symptoms that suggest hypoglycaemia or hyperglycaemia. Therefore, there is a critical need to examine the analytical and clinical accuracy of the measured glucose levels obtained by such commercial glucose meters. The analytical accuracy can be described as the deviation between the reference and measured values. This parameter alone is not sufficient for the task of monitoring patients' SMBG errors and the clinical consequence. This chapter addresses analytical accuracy and clinical accuracy of SMBG errors and compares the new type 1 diabetes error grid with a traditional Clarke error grid. Thus, it is important to consider if an improvement in analytical accuracy would lead to improved clinical outcomes for patients.

Surprisingly, there are several scenarios where analytical tools used in the description of SMBG with accuracy could be irrelevant to treatment decisions.

Keywords: self-monitoring blood glucose; analytical accuracy; clinical accuracy; error grid

CONTENTS

INTRODUCTION

Systems or devices for self-monitoring of blood glucose have advanced significantly during the last 50 years; however, they are still based on glucose oxidase, a very stable and specific enzyme for the oxidation of glucose to D–gluconolactone. This is an oxygen-dependent enzyme, so the determination can be followed by oxygen consumption or the formation of hydrogen peroxide. The measurement is also vulnerable to endogenous species such as ascorbic acid, uric acid and other electroactive compounds including drugs and their metabolites. The second enzyme, glucose dehydrogenase, is oxygen independent but a co-enzyme, β-NAD(H), is needed in this reaction. Strictly speaking, there is no reference method for the assay of glucose in the central laboratory, but the hexokinase is widely accepted in various hospital and clinical settings. Detailed information concerning the components of currently available SMBG systems is limited, and the accuracy and standardised reporting of SMBG devices remain a key concern. Intensive therapy of type 1 diabetes with insulin reduces the risks of new-onset retinopathy and retards retinopathy progression very significantly. For noninsulin-treated type 2 diabetes, the role of SMBG is somewhat controversial. Patients subject to the following treatment/ condition are also tested for their glucose levels: parenteral hyperalimentation, medications affecting blood glucose concentration, liver or pancreas operation, post-operation or post-procedure elevations in glucose secondary to stress with infection, and undergoing renal dialysis. This chapter addresses the analytical accuracy, measurement errors and clinical accuracy of SMBG and its role in diabetic therapy.

LACK OF A STANDARD METHOD FOR GLUCOSE MEASUREMENT

Analytical accuracy compares the result of a measurement by a glucose device with a measurement by a reference method for this assay. To date, there is no internationally accepted reference method for the measurement of blood glucose. In the past, the Centers for Disease Control and Prevention (CDC) recommended a method based on isotope dilution gas chromatography–mass spectrometry (IDGC-MS) as a standard method for glucose measurement. The method involved the dilution of the sample with an isotope of glucose and measured in a gas chromatograph equipped with mass spectrometry.[1] Also, no universal reference material works on all glucose measuring systems and the matrix effect from sample to sample is always problematic.[2] Two reference procedures have been commonly used for glucose measurement: hexokinase (HK) glucose-6-phosphate dehydrogenase (G6PD), and glucose oxidase (GOD)-peroxidase. In some cases, GOD-oxygen electrode and GOD-dry chemistry are also used. Therefore, different methods and instruments often lead to variations in results from laboratory to laboratory.[3] Routine HK methods show a higher accuracy than GOD methods, but two measurement systems meet the minimal quality specifications. The reference materials for glucose measurement with the highest metrological level are available at the American National Institute of Standards and Technology (NIST), but their high cost and difficulty of transportation limit the widespread use of such materials for assessment and validation.[4] However, the reference serum total protein can be prepared as recommended by the American Association for Clinical Chemistry (AACC).

EFFECT OF PARTIAL PRESSURE OF OXYGEN IN BLOOD SAMPLES

The pO2 level in capillary blood samples is 70 mmHg[5] and might be lower in patients with respiratory diseases or higher if they receive oxygen therapy. Most of the self-monitoring glucose devices use glucose oxidase, an oxygen-dependent enzyme for the oxidation of glucose. Considering the glucose value obtained at 70 mmHg as the mean, various GOD systems might have mean relative differences between 11.8% and 44.5% at pO2 values below 45 mmHg and between −14.6% and −21.2% at pO2 values above 150 mmHg. The magnitude of the pO2 effect also varies among these systems. As mentioned in Chapter 2, some manufacturers might incorporate a glucose diffusion limiting membrane to overcome the oxygen effect. Other systems rely on an electron acceptor (mediator), such as ferrocene, ferricyanide, or a conducting organic salt to minimise the oxygen dependency, and the detection can be performed at low applied potentials to minimise electroactive interference. Consequently, a diabetic person might have two or more meters at home with different calibration and readings. As expected for the system with glucose dehydrogenase, such values are only −0.3% and −0.2%, respectively, at such two extreme pO2 because oxygen does not participate in this reaction. Therefore, the pO2 effect and range should be provided in the product information. Otherwise, blood glucose values can be over- or underestimated, resulting in undetected hypo- or hyperglycaemic events. Of course, other factors must be considered as temperature, haematocrit, and interfering drugs also exhibit a noticeable influence on blood glucose measurements.

Glucose oxidase-mediator biosensor strips are often sensitive to oxygen concentration as both the mediator and oxygen compete to take electrons from the reduced form of glucose oxidase ($FADH_2$). Only the mediator is detected by the electrode; the sample with a high oxygen content will result in an underestimated value and vice versa. Therefore, the glucose oxidase strip precalibrated with capillary blood is most accurate in SMBG with capillary blood. The glucose dehydrogenase system is not affected by oxygen, but this enzyme presents other limitations. In brief, galactose, xylose and maltose compete with glucose on glucose dehydrogenase and result in false values.

INTERFERENCE AND INTERFERING SPECIES

As mentioned in other chapters, some endogenous species in blood samples might cause interference, leading to falsely high or falsely low values.

Ascorbic acid

This electroactive compound can provoke an interference with both

GOD and GDH-FAD-based electrochemical strips by oxidisation at the electrode surface, resulting in falsely elevated blood glucose readings.[6] Ascorbic acid as high as 1–5 M can be achieved by the intravenous route as an alternate or adjuvant to chemotherapy or radiotherapy. This prooxidant generates hydrogen peroxide-dependent selective cytotoxicity to cancer cells *in vitro*.[7] Considering its half-life of 2.0 ±0.6 h,[8] one has to wait at least 8–10 h after intravenous ascorbic acid to perform glucose monitoring with GOD strips. The hexokinase procedure is not affected by ascorbic acid.

Triglycerides

They are not electroactive but their presence usually at very high levels will take up the volume, and so decrease the amount of glucose in the capillary volume. Thus, the reading of glucose is inaccurate and low.

Uric acid

This acid can cause falsely high values only at very high concentrations and is seldom a problem, except in patients with severe gout.[9]

Temperature

This effect is seldom a problem except for mountain climbers who are subject to extreme temperatures. At 8 °C, the errors of the measured glucose level can be ± 5–7%.[10] However, low temperature diminishes circulation to the skin; the blood flow to the skin of the forearm is significantly decreased. Glucose taken from a fingertip is not affected significantly since the arteriovenous shunts of the fingers stay open. However, strips exposed to 40 °C for several months can provoke falsely higher glucose values since the oxidised mediator used in the strip is somewhat unstable and can be reduced, particularly at high temperature.[11] Such test strips when tested for glucose samples at 110 mg/dL reported significantly higher values, even as high as 300 mg/dL.

Haematocrit

Variation in haematocrit might cause significant errors in blood glucose when measured by SMBG. Blood has two major components: plasma and cells; and the percentage of red cells is the haematocrit, which contains significant amounts of intracellular glucose.[12] Glucose in erythrocytes is in equilibrium with plasma glucose but at lower levels. This variation is due solely to the altered contribution of the RBC to the whole blood value. The total blood glucose, therefore, is dependent on the haematocrit. Although some glucose meters use intricate systems to evaluate haematocrit and correct for it, the effect of haematocrit is more complex. The cells contain glucose at a different concentration than plasma and can block the enzyme on the test strip and provoke errors as large as 40% at very low haematocrit.[13]

ANALYTICAL ACCURACY IN CLINICALLY ILL PATIENTS

Among several glucose meters tested, the best group has inaccuracies of 5.5–7%, the slightly less accurate group with inaccuracies of 7–8.5%, and the least accurate with inaccuracies greater than 8.5%. All companies have tested their systems and provide both the inaccuracy figures and the ISO numbers. However, the level of accuracy is expected to approach over 95% with newer and advanced technologies. According to ISO 15197-2013 (E), also known as 'in vitro diagnostic test systems requirements for blood glucose monitoring systems for self-testing in managing diabetes mellitus', the required accuracy is as follows: 95% of the measured glucose values shall fall within ± 15 mg/dL of the average measured values of the reference measurement procedure at glucose concentrations < 100 mg/dL or within ± 15% at glucose concentrations ≥ 100 mg/dL. Also 99% of individual glucose measured values shall fall within zones A and B of the Clarke error grid for type 1 diabetes as discussed later. In hospital settings, 99% of all values obtained by the device must be within a range of ± 10% of the reference method for glucose concentrations > 70 mg/dL and within ± 7 mg/dL at glucose concentrations < 70 mg/dL.

A study of 152 patients who were experienced in SMBG revealed that only 45% of the patients' measurements were within 10% of the hexokinase value, and only 63% were within 15%.[13] In addition, the accuracy of blood glucose measurements using glucose meters and arterial blood gas analysers in critically ill adult patients is very disturbing. Blood glucose measurements in the hypoglycaemic range are less accurate than are those in the normal range and, in some cases, the result is outside the agreement range up to 38%.[14] Inaccuracy is not related to the patients' sex, body mass index, the severity of illness, and the presence of sepsis and/or diabetes. A glucose meter using arterial blood is significantly more accurate than a glucose meter using capillary blood in critically ill patients. Among 6000 samples tested for the accuracy of blood glucose measurements, only 70 samples were in the hypoglycaemic range. Therefore, further assessments are needed for blood glucose measurements in the very high range. Also, unstable haemodynamics and insulin infusion were associated with increased risk of inaccuracy. Apparently, current blood glucose monitoring devices lack a high degree of accuracy and reliability for glucose monitoring and control in critically ill patients. More systematic studies are still needed to improve the accuracy of blood glucose monitoring devices and eliminate sources of error. In addition, acetaminophen, L-DOPA, tolazamide, and ascorbic acid are well known to interfere with the glucose oxidase system whereas icodextrin, a component of some peritoneal dialysis fluids, interferes with glucose dehydrogenase.

CLINICAL ACCURACY AND THE CLARKE ERROR GRID

An error grid, also known as the Clarke grid, was created by a group of investigators from the University of Virginia as shown in Fig. 7.1.[15,16] In brief, each point on the grid (true blood glucose (BG), measured BG) is associated with one of five risk levels: **A**: SMBG 20% deviation from true BG or both SMBG and BG 70 mg/dL, **B**: deviation from true BG 20% but no treatment or only benign treatment, **C**: overcorrection of acceptable BG levels, **D**: dangerous failure to detect and treat BG errors, and **E**: erroneous treatment. This grid chart signifies the clinical importance of SMBG errors and has been widely accepted.[17–19] This elegant method was innovative because it considered the difference between the system-generated and reference blood glucose values as well as the clinical significance of such a difference.

However, continuous glucose–error grid analysis (CG-EGA) is very time-consuming because the accuracy assessment requires frequent blood sampling. This could be more problematic for its applicability to assess novel glucose devices with large-scale investigations.

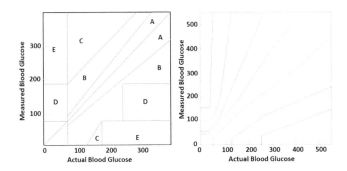

FIGURE 7.1 The SMBG data from the clinical trial superimposed on the error grid of Clarke et al. (A) and on the type 1 diabetes error grid (B). (Reproduced with permission from the American Diabetes Association.[13])

The Clarke EGA only evaluates the correspondence and discrepancy between sensor readings and blood glucose values at isolated static points in time. It does not consider the relationship of data points as a function of time. In continuous monitoring systems, data at a given point are related to those nearby to indicate the trend in glucose variation. The Clarke error grid was also scrutinised by a consortium of 100 endocrinologists and the SMBG data from the clinical trial is plotted on both the Clarke error grid (Fig. 7.1A) and the new error grid for type 1 diabetes (Fig. 7.1B). In brief, most (98.6%) of the measurements are As or Bs on the new grid compared to 95% on the Clarke grid, due to the modification of the abrupt A/B and B/D boundaries on the Clarke grid that reflects advanced glucose devices for SMBG. The new chart shown in Fig. 7.1A-B is also more tolerant to SMBG errors, and the new chart eliminates the entire high glucose E zone.

In conclusion, an intense treatment regime can reduce the risk of nephropathy, retinopathy, and neuropathy up to 70% for type 1 diabetic patients[20] and type 2 diabetes.[3,21,22] However, the patients must monitor their blood glucose at least 3 or 4 times per day. There is still a need for a gold standard for glucose measurement and the reference material for glucose must be more affordable and available. Diabetes is on the rise due to the lifestyle changes of modern society and it is a great challenge to control this disease. Diabetes therapy requires the accurate monitoring of blood glucose levels in the central laboratory as well as the accuracy of self-monitoring of blood glucose levels. Newer and more advanced technology enables the manufacturer to provide test strips with minimal variation. Such strips are dependent on the quality of the electrodes and the distribution of the enzyme-mediator on the sensing area. The maximum lot-to-lot difference among test strips should be less than 1.0%, and such strips normally have an excess amount of the enzyme and the mediator to ensure that moderate loss of these components during storage or other abused conditions does not significantly affect the reading.

REFERENCES

1. Björkhem I, Blomstrand R, Falk O, Öhman G. The use of mass fragmentography in the evaluation of routine methods for glucose determination. *Clin Chim Acta.* 1976; 72(3): 353–62.
2. Hagvik J. Glucose measurement: time for a gold standard. *J Diabetes Sci Technol.* 2007; 1(2): 169–72.
3. Gambino R. Glucose: a simple molecule that is not simple to quantify. *Clin Chem.* 2007; 53(12): 2040–1.

4. Xia C, Liu O, Wang L, Xu G. Trueness assessment for serum glucose measurement using commercial systems through the preparation of commutable reference materials. *Ann Lab Med.* 2012; 32(4): 243–9.

5. Higgins C. Capillary blood gases: to arterialize or not. *MLO Med Lab Obs.* 2008; 40(42): 4–7.

6. Tang Z, Du X, Louie RF, Kost GJ. Effects of drugs on glucose measurements with handheld glucose meters and a portable glucose analyzer. *Am J Clin Pathol.* 2000; 113(1): 75–86.

7. Chen Q, Espey MG, Krishna MC, Mitchell JB, Corpe CP, Buettner GR, et al. Pharmacologic ascorbic acid concentrations selectively kill cancer cells: action as a pro-drug to deliver hydrogen peroxide to tissues. *Proc Natl Acad Sci USA.* 2005; 102(38): 13604–9.

8. Stephenson CM, Levin RD, Spector T, Lis CG. Phase I clinical trial to evaluate the safety, tolerability, and pharmacokinetics of high-dose intravenous ascorbic acid in patients with advanced cancer. *Cancer Chemother Pharmacol.* 2013; 72(1): 139–46.

9. Bishop ML, Duben-Engelkirk JL, Fody EP. *Clinical Chemistry: Principles, Procedures, Correlations.* Lippincott Williams & Wilkins; 2000.

10. Ginsberg BH. Factors affecting blood glucose monitoring: sources of errors in measurement. *J Diabetes Sci Technol.* 2009; 3(4): 903–13.

11. Bamberg R, Schulman K, MacKenzie M, Moore J, Olchesky S. Effect of adverse storage conditions on performance of glucometer test strips. *Clin Lab Sci.* 2005; 18(4): 203–9.

12. Somogyi M. The distribution of sugar in normal human blood. *J Biol Chem.* 1928; 78(1): 117–27.

13. Parkes JL, Slatin SL, Pardo S, Ginsberg BH. A new consensus error grid to evaluate the clinical significance of inaccuracies in the measurement of blood glucose. *Diabetes Care.* 2000; 23(8): 1143–8.

14. Inoue S, Egi M, Kotani J, Morita K. Accuracy of blood-glucose measurements using glucose meters and arterial blood gas analyzers in critically ill adult patients: systematic review. *Crit Care.* 2013; 17(2): R48.

15. Clarke WL, Cox D, Gonder-Frederick LA, Carter W, Pohl SL. Evaluating clinical accuracy of systems for self-monitoring of blood glucose. *Diabetes Care.* 1987; 10(5): 622–8.

16. Cox DJ, Clarke WL, Gonder-Frederick L, Pohl S, Hoover C, Snyder A, et al. Accuracy of perceiving blood glucose in IDDM. *Diabetes Care.* 1985; 8(6): 529–36.

17. Brunner GA, Ellmerer M, Sendlhofer G, Wutte A, Trajanoski Z, Schaupp L, et al. Validation of home blood glucose meters with respect to clinical and analytical approaches. *Diabetes Care.* 1998; 21(4): 585–90.

18. Trajanoski Z, Brunner GA, Schaupp L, Ellmerer M, Wach P, Pieber TR, et al. Open-flow microperfusion of subcutaneous adipose tissue for on-line continuous *ex vivo* measurement of glucose concentration. *Diabetes Care.* 1997; 20(7): 1114–21.

19. O'Brien PC, Wise SD, Ness S, LeBlanc SM. Dermal interstitial glucose as an indicator of ambient glycemia. *Diabetes Care.* 1997; 20(9): 1426–9.

20. The Diabetes Control and Complications Trial Research Group. The effect of intensive treatment of diabetes on the development and progression of long-term complications in insulin-dependent diabetes mellitus. *N Engl J Med.* 1993; 329(14): 977–86.

21. American Diabetes Association. Standards of medical care in diabetes – 2013. *Diabetes Care.* 2013; 36(Suppl 1): S11.

22. UK Prospective Diabetes Study Group. Intensive blood-glucose control with sulphonylureas or insulin compared with conventional treatment and risk of complications in patients with type 2 diabetes (UKPDS 33). *Lancet.* 1998; 352(9131): 837–53.

CHAPTER 8

Concluding remarks

Sandeep Kumar Vashist and John HT Luong

The American adult population with diabetes is estimated to be 12% while over a third of those aged 20 and above might have prediabetes.[1] In China, there are 114 million people with diabetes and 493 million people with prediabetes.[2] The diabetes epidemic is also on the rise in India. In 2013, 67 million people in India are confirmed to have diabetes with another 30 million having prediabetes.[3] The situation in Saudi Arabia is very serious concerning this country's looming diabetes disaster. One in four Saudis is very likely to suffer a heart attack, and diabetes is the leading cause of cardiovascular disease.[4] The report also revealed that more than 60% of diabetics die of a heart attack. Diabetes also brings other complications such as gestational diabetes, diabetic foot ulcers and heart diseases. In the US alone, the total cost of diagnosed diabetes was about $245 billion in 2013, a substantial burden on society.[5]

Glucose monitoring is the first step in diabetes control and management and also plays a major role in prediabetes with people who need to return their blood sugar back to normal with healthy diet and physical exercise. As diabetics need to test their blood glucose levels daily, glucose is the most commonly tested analyte and dominates the entire biosensor market. Biosensor technology has come a long way since Clark and Lyons pioneered the initial concept in 1962 (Table 8.1). Intensive research on new sensing concepts and novel materials, coupled with advanced fabrication, has resulted in several elegant devices being commercially available for the self-testing of glucose. After several generations of improvement, daily testing of blood glucose still suffers from low and irregular testing frequency due to the inconvenience and discomfort of the test.

Glucose fluctuation is still a major concern for patients with type 1 diabetes since blood glucose levels can swing between low and high from 2–3 mM to over 20 mM within a day and unpredictable trends and patterns. Therefore, diabetic patients must perform their glucose measurement several times a day. Unfortunately, intermittent testing performed eight times a day still misses the episodes of such extreme glucose fluctuations. The practice of finger pricking is the only option, but cannot be applied during sleep or while driving or doing other urgent daily activities. It is hard to fathom how it could be achieved if the patient is a police officer, pilot or firefighter!

More frequent measurements or continuous monitoring provides maximal information about daily blood glucose levels, the trend, duration and frequency of fluctuations.[6] Therefore, the ultimate goal is the development of non-invasive glucose sensing for continuous glucose monitoring to eliminate pain and discomfort associated with daily testing. This approach has been extended towards glucose measurements in sweat, saliva or tears. Urine tests are never used to diagnose diabetes, but the levels of urine ketones and urine glucose are good indicators of whether the diabetes is being managed well.

A needle-type electrode can be subcutaneously implanted for continuous monitoring of glucose in the interstitial fluid. Although functional, the measurement lags behind the true blood glucose concentration after a meal when glycemia is changing rapidly. This concept has been commercialised with limited success since the measurement only lasts for 3–4 days and the system must be calibrated 3–4 times a day against conventional finger pricking. Other technical issues include electrode fouling, varying tissue $pO2$, tissue interfering species, etc. that affect the electrode reading, meaning the system must be calibrated very frequently.

A different approach is to implant a hollow dialysis fibre to get glucose from the tissue and pump it outside the body for measurement by a conventional glucose meter. Microdialysis has been commercialised by several companies; however, more clinical trials are still needed to validate its clinical potential and analytical accuracy. Glucose obtained by microdialysis can induce a decrease in viscosity of dextran bound to Concanavalin A (Con A), and this concept has been developed by Disetronic/Roche as the viscometric glucose sensor.[7] In brief, glucose binds strongly to Con A to liberate dextran, prebound to Con A, and the resulting viscosity change can be measured by a pressure transducer.

Considerable efforts also continue towards the development of chronically implanted devices to improve the control and management of diabetes. GlySens[8] is reported to develop a truly long-term continuous glucose monitoring system. The device is expected to have

1 year or longer life, and it has been demonstrated up to 18 months in preclinical studies. However, the patient needs a short outpatient procedure to insert the sensor probably in the lower abdomen area, with an expected operating life of 1 year or longer. This is a glucose-specific, oxygen-based, dual-enzyme electrode technology, adapted from the standard laboratory method. However, its availability is not imminent as the device must be subject to a larger human trial and FDA regulatory filing/approval. It should be noted that two competing companies, Dexcom and Medtronic, have turned their attention away from long-term implantable sensors. The next major challenge is the connection of the device to a closed-loop system for optimal insulin delivery. Other considerable hurdles include the body's rejection, the sensor's long-term stability, oxygen limitation, miniaturisation, and infection. Doubtlessly, the ultimate implementation of the new glucose devices is dictated by commercial and legal considerations, not scientific breakthroughs or achievements, unless the issues mentioned above can be resolved in the most effective and elegant way. Nevertheless, the GlucoWatch® Biographer (Cygnus, Inc.) is a wristwatch that provides glucose measurements non-invasively through the skin every 20 min for up to 12 h at a time. After a 3-h warm-up period, the GlucoWatch® Biographer is calibrated using a fingerstick measurement and ready for monitoring glucose values. Together with fingerstick glucose measurements, it provides additional glucose information about glucose trends and patterns.

Direct oxidation of glucose without the enzyme deserves a brief comment here since this 'enzymeless' approach is not vulnerable to pH, temperature, etc. and circumvents the use of glucose oxidase in *in vivo* monitoring. Considerable attention has focused on platinum-based electrodes for direct oxidation of glucose in neutral media. Various strategies have been advocated to improve the detection sensitivity such as bimetallic/polymetallic platinum-based nanomaterials, and effective supports for nano-sized platinum loading. Although some obtained results are encouraging, this approach has been tested for 'very clean' samples, not blood per se. Various species in the blood can be adsorbed onto the platinum surface and are electrochemically active; that is, they can be oxidised or reduced to interfere with the detection of glucose. Such well-known species include ascorbic acid, uric acid, dopamine, etc. Other sugars such as fructose and galactose are expected to cause significant interference. Electrode fouling or poisoning is another drawback of this approach since amino acids and blood-based proteins also strongly adhere to the platinum surface. Adsorption of intermediates and products during the glucose electrooxidation process is another technical issue that needs to be addressed. To date, this approach remains as an academic curiosity.

The development of fluorescence-based glucose sensors is another research topic because this approach might offer some unique advantages for biological analysis. Besides concanavalin A (Con A), several receptors have been employed to detect glucose in fluorescence sensors. Various fluorophores are useful for the sensitive detection of hydrogen peroxide, the by-product of glucose oxidation by glucose oxidase. However, the requirement of such added fluorophores prevents the practical application of this approach for glucose sensing by diabetics. To date, fluorescence-based biosensors have not entered clinical practice in diabetes management. Nevertheless, the intrinsic fluorescence of skin (NAD(P)H) might offer a non-invasive approach to *in vivo* glucose monitoring. In our body system, several glucose-dependent pathways are known to generate the fluorescent cofactor NADP(H) from non-fluorescent NAD(P).

Lastly, the glucose device must be combined with another detection scheme for a diabetic biomarker. Besides glycated haemoglobin, as discussed in this book, fructosamine, glycated albumin (GA), and 1,5-anhydroglucitol (1,5-AG) should be considered to complement the limitations of the glycated haemoglobin assay. In particular, 1,5-AG might serve as an indicator for estimating within-day glucose variation. There is also a link between obesity, inflammation and insulin resistance that indicates the important secretory role of adipose tissue. Cytokines and adipokines synthesised by enlarged adipose tissue are related to impaired glucose metabolism. Thus, it is of importance to develop standardised automated assay methods for these novel biomarkers as useful prognostic factors for diabetes and its complications.

Diabetic patients always monitor and keep a close watch on their glucose concentrations, but they do not measure and are unaware of their insulin levels. To prevent 'hypoglycaemia', the liver continuously makes glucose and transports it into the blood even during fasting. Thus, the glucose balance is maintained by circulating insulin, whose level should never be zero except for a person with untreated type 1 diabetes. In contrast, a high level of insulin can be problematic, an indicator of insulin resistance, prediabetes, or early-stage type 2 diabetes. Elevated insulin promotes insulin resistance, lowers magnesium levels, and increases inflammation. It also tends to decrease HDL ('good') cholesterol and raises levels of LDL ('bad') cholesterol, leading to heart disease.

A fasting insulin level test is also valuable in the differentiation of type 2 from latent autoimmune diabetes of adults (LADA). A person with type 2 might have a normal or even high fasting insulin level whereas a person with LADA has typically low fasting insulin level. Thus, a person with LADA is more likely to benefit from insulin injection, avoiding years of oral medications with low positive outcomes. The test also plays an important role to ascertain if a person diagnosed with type 1 diabetes is still making some insulin considering the fact that about three-quarters of adults with type 1 produce small amounts of insulin.

The measurement of insulin is more challenging and complicated, compared to glucose monitoring. In brief, insulin, a peptide hormone, inhibits the production of glucose by the liver. It also promotes the absorption of glucose from the blood to skeletal muscles and fat tissue, rendering fat to be stored rather than used for energy. Different immunoassay formats have been developed for insulin owing to the availability of insulin antibody. Indeed, micromethods for the assay of insulin based on the reaction between ^{131}I-labelled insulin and insulin antibody were developed in the early 1960s and Dr Rosalyn S Yalow received the Nobel Prize for this wonderful development.[9] Modern immunoassays are based on a labeled enzyme, such as horseradish peroxidase (HRP), and a sandwich assay format. The capture antibody is conjugated to a solid substrate (surface), which 'captures' insulin to form a stable complex. The enzyme-labelled antibody then forms a tertiary complex with the insulin-capture antibody complex. The labelled enzyme, such as HRP, catalyses tetramethylbenzidine, one of the most sensitive chromogenic substrates, in the presence of hydrogen peroxide and the reaction can be followed by measuring the absorbance of the yellow product at 450 nm.

Direct electrochemical measurements of insulin are of considerable interest in connection with the development of glucose sensing for monitoring insulin secretion and therapeutic insulin formulations. The measurement, however, is limited because of the slow kinetics of insulin oxidation at common electrode materials. Insulin is a simple protein (MW = 5730 Da) with a known structure. Insulin has two chains (A and B) with three disulfide bonds; two are interchain (A7B7 and A20B19), and one is an intrachain bond (A6A11). The A7B7, located on the surface of the insulin molecule, is very accessible. The A20B19 is somewhat accessible whereas the A6A11 is least reactive. Therefore, electrochemistry of insulin involves the breakage of the A7B7 and A20B19 disulfide bonds.[10] Electrodes have been chemically modified for promoting the oxidation and detection of insulin, with limited success. Of interest is the electropolymerisation of rhodamine B in the presence of carbon nanotube on a glassy carbon electrode. The resulting electrode exhibits a linear dynamic range of 100–600 nM with a detection limit of 5 nM.[11] More detailed studies are needed to assess the performance of electrochemical sensing in the different blood samples.

In clinical diagnosis, the average insulin level in the US is expressed as 8.8 mIU/mL for men and 8.4 mIU/mL for women. However, the ideal level of fasting insulin should be well below 8.4 mIU/mL and one unit of insulin is equal to 0.0347 mg. In the past, one unit was defined as the amount of insulin that will lower the blood glucose of a healthy and fasting rabbit for 24 h to 2.5 mM (45 mg/dL) within 5 h. U100 is the most common type of insulin, 100 units of insulin in 1 mL of solution. Diabetic patients, particularly type 1, also need to have the anti-insulin antibody test checks to see if their bodies have produced antibodies against insulin. If the test is positive for IgG and IgM antibodies against insulin, their bodies identify insulin as foreign matter. Thus, treatment with insulin becomes less or not effective. Another complication includes skin reactions at the site of the insulin injection, which might require desensitisation.

The last word for non-invasive technology is exciting news from a company in Israel that combines three independent technologies: ultrasonic, electromagnetic and thermal, to painlessly obtain blood glucose levels in the ear lobe. The measurement is not of the blood directly, but the technology is based on the measurement of a range of physiological phenomena within the body, which are correlated with glucose levels.[12] This is different from optical technology, which has long been pursued by several companies for non-invasive blood glucose monitoring. Glucowise technology enables the blood glucose concentration to be measured at the capillary level, unlike the standard optical methods that measure glucose at the level of the skin or use other body fluids such as interstitial fluid.[13] Hopefully, diabetic patients can purchase such devices soon since they have been waiting for so long for a breakthrough development. There has been a plethora of 'breaking news' over the last 20 years without any real device in the market to enable a viable non-invasive or painless technique with reliable and accurate measurement of glucose.

The message is clear: as the tools for monitoring and controlling blood glucose have improved, the number of people with diabetic complications has decreased. However, the patient with diabetes has to keep blood sugar levels stable. Lifestyle changes and diet balance are no longer an option, and this is a balancing act.

TABLE 8.1 Progress and improvement in biosensor technology for glucose sensing

Type of devices	General performance and characteristics
First generation	• Glucose oxidase together with an oxygen probe or a metal electrode (platinum) for hydrogen peroxide determination. For the latter, a permselective coating is implemented to minimise electroactive interfering species. Electropolymerised films of poly-(phenylenediamine), polyphenol, and overoxidised polypyrrole have been widely used and found effective. Other coatings involve size exclusion cellulose acetate films, Nafion, Kodak AQ ionomers, alkanethiol or lipid layers or their combination. This limitation of oxygen (known as the 'oxygen deficit') can be overcome by using diffusion-limiting films of polycarbonate or polyurethane to increase the oxygen/glucose permeability ratio.
Second generation	• Artificial mediators are used to shuttle electrons between the FAD centre of glucose oxidase and the electrode surface. Common mediators are ferricyanide, ferrocene derivatives, conducting organic salts, quinones, transition-metal complexes, etc. Commercial glucose devices use ferricyanide or ferrocene mediators. This concept is very limited to *in vivo* applications due to potential leaching, instability, and toxicity of the mediator for an extended operation.
	• Enzyme wiring with a redox polymer, e.g. poly(vinylpyridine) or poly(vinylimidazole), with a dense array of osmium-complex electron relays. The redox polymer binds the enzyme to form a three-dimensional network that reduces the distance between the polymer redox centre and the FAD centre of glucose oxidase.
	• Modification of glucose oxidase with electron-relay groups of ferrocene-monocarboxylic acid to the enzyme.
	• Modification of glucose oxidase with electron relays and obtaining an efficient electrical contact. The enzyme FAD active centre can be removed to allow positioning of an electron-mediating ferrocene unit. The resulting complex is reconstituted with the apoenzyme (FAD-minus).
	• Nanoparticles and carbon nanotubes can be used as electrical connectors between the electrode and the enzyme redox centre.
Third generation	• The electron is transferred directly from glucose to the electrode via the enzyme active site. This is an active and somewhat controversial research area with several conflicting reports. Different electrode materials, particularly boron-doped diamond electrodes, display direct electron transfer with glucose oxidase.

REFERENCES

1. Diabetes rise in the US is 'alarming,' say CDC. www.medicalnewstoday com/articles/278140php. 2014.
2. Caring for diabetes in China. www.diabetesforecastorg/2015/jan-feb/ caring-diabetes-chinahtml. 2015.
3. Diabetes epidemic on the rise in India. http://timesofindiaindiatimescom/ life-style/health-fitness/health-news/Diabetes-epidemic-on-the-rise-in-India/articleshow/25758884cms. 2013.
4. Sarant L. Saudi Arabia's looming diabetes disaster. *NatureMiddleEast.* doi: 10.1038/nmiddleeast.2015.35
5. The cost of diabetes. www.diabetesorg/advocacy/news-events/cost-of-diabeteshtml?referrer=https://wwwgooglecoil/. 2013.
6. Pickup JC, Hussain F, Evans ND, Sachedina N. *In vivo* glucose monitoring: the clinical reality and the promise. *Biosens Bioelectron.* 2005; 20(10): 1897–902.
7. Beyer U, Schafer D, Thomas A, Aulich H, Haueter U, Reihl B, et al. Recording of subcutaneous glucose dynamics by a viscometric affinity sensor. *Diabetologia.* 2001; 44(4): 416–23.
8. GlySens. http://glysens.com/. 2014.
9. Yalow RS. Radioimmunoassay: a probe for fine structure of biologic systems. Nobel Lecture, 8 December, 1977. www.nobelprize.org/nobel_prizes/medicine/laureates/1977/yalow-lecture.pdf.
10. Stankovich MA, Bard A. The electrochemistry of proteins and related substances. Part II. Insulin. *J Electroanl Chem.* 1977; 85: 173–83.
11. Hatefi–Mehrjardia A, Karimi MA, Kamalabadi-Khorasani S. Rhodamine B–multi-walled carbon nanotubes modified glassy carbon electrode. *Procedia Materials Sci.* 2015; 11: 162–5.
12. www.medgadget.com/2013/10/non-invasive-measurement-of-blood-glucose-levels-using-glucotrack-interview.html?trendmd-shared=0.
13. www.gluco-wise.com.

Index

Entries in **bold** denote tables; entries in *italics* denote figures.